Over the course of about two years, she lost over one hundred fifty pounds through hard work and slow but steady progress. Linda is a total love…incredibly honest, humble, and generous, and 110 percent committed to helping others get healthy. She's also a very talented writer.

—Joy Bauer, MS, RD, CDN
Nutrition and Health Expert for *The Today Show*

I have known Linda for many years, and while her body may have shrunk, her heart has enlarged! Her passion and desire is for others to get healthier mentally, physically, and spiritually, and she has proven that it doesn't take rocket science or a fat wallet to feel better. With common sense Linda will open your eyes to the possibilities of change and help you see a brighter, slimmer and healthier future. She has successfully proven that you can be the person you've always wanted to be!

—Donna VanLiere
New York Times Best-Selling Author

You will love Linda's vulnerability! As an expert in the field of sexuality, I'm constantly counseling women whose appetite for intimacy is crucified by their appetites for chili-cheese fries…only they don't realize it. Linda doesn't just offer you the key to a better budget and waistline in this delightfully written book, she's offering you the key to unlock your passion with your spouse again. And she's not afraid to talk about it.

—Dannah Gresh
Author of *What Are You Waiting For: The One Thing No One Ever Tells You About Sex* and *The Bride Wore White*, and Coauthor of *Lies Young Women Believe*

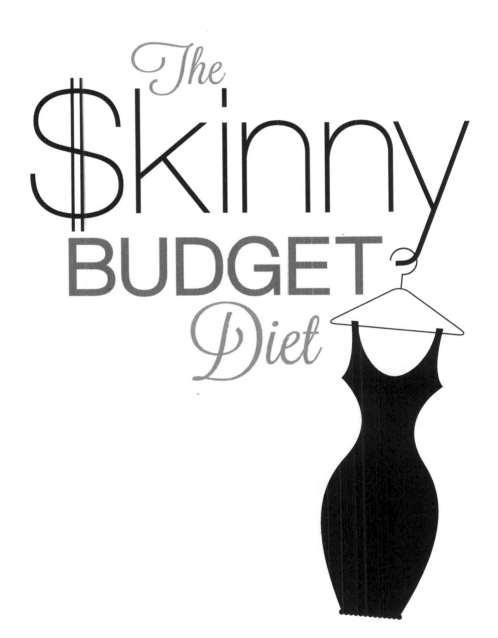

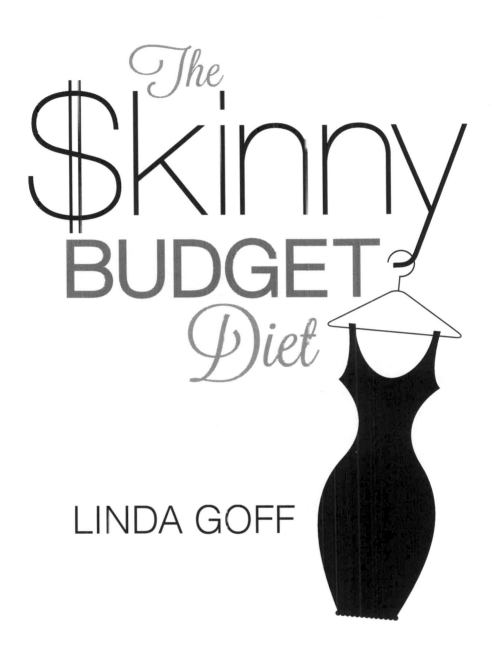

The $kinny BUDGET Diet

LINDA GOFF

SILOAM

Most CHARISMA HOUSE BOOK GROUP products are available at special quantity discounts for bulk purchase for sales promotions, premiums, fund-raising, and educational needs. For details, write Charisma House Book Group, 600 Rinehart Road, Lake Mary, Florida 32746, or telephone (407) 333-0600.

THE SKINNY BUDGET DIET by Linda Goff
Published by Siloam
Charisma Media/Charisma House Book Group
600 Rinehart Road
Lake Mary, Florida 32746
www.charismahouse.com

Unless otherwise noted, all Scripture quotations are from the Holy Bible, New International Version. Copyright © 1973, 1978, 1984, International Bible Society. Used by permission.

Scripture quotations marked KJV are from the King James Version of the Bible.

Scripture quotations marked NKJV are from the New King James Version of the Bible. Copyright © 1979, 1980, 1982 by Thomas Nelson, Inc., publishers. Used by permission.

Cover design by Nancy Panaccione
Design Director: Bill Johnson

Visit the author's website at www.theskinnybudgetdiet.com.

Library of Congress Cataloging-in-Publication Data:
An application to register this book for cataloging has been submitted
to the Library of Congress.
International Standard Book Number: 978-1-62136-001-8
E-book ISBN: 978-1-62136-002-5

13 14 15 16 17 — 9 8 7 6 5 4 3 2
Printed in the United States of America

Dedication

To my husband, Dan, and my sons,
Alex and Nathan...the guys who
loved me through thick and thin

To my Lord Jesus...a Savior who
loved me enough to die for me

CONTENTS

Acknowledgments

Special thanks to:

Margie Shealy with the Christian Medical and Dental Associations; Rita Hancock, MD; Steve Hanor, MD; Nick Yphantides, MD; Mary Bruns, DO; Blythe Daniel; Greentree Christian Church; my faithful Brown clan cheerleaders (Edward, Claire, and Karen); and my brave friends who encouraged me to write this book. You have enriched my life in more ways than I could ever count.

Introduction

LIVING HIGH ON THE HOG

IN THE TIME it took me to grow from a two-hundred-pound college student into a three-hundred-pound mother of two, I learned a few things. Thanksgiving turkeys shouldn't be cooked to medium rare. Don't mix ammonia and bleach in the same toilet. And if you are going to eat five thousand calories a day, buy sturdy furniture. Good stuff to know that I didn't learn in school.

All of the hours I spent studying literature, chemistry, and physics would have been better spent in a class called Math and Science for Life. The entire semester would be focused on these simple rules: Watch your pennies, and the dollars will take care of themselves. Watch your calories, and the pounds will take care of themselves.

If you struggle with your weight, I'm guessing that calorie counting isn't something on your daily to-do list. It wasn't on mine. And although it may seem like a separate issue, I think we must also ask: How is the money adding up? Do you know how much money you spend every month? Do you feel like you are steering your budget or just reacting to the bill that must be paid today or else?

It is ironic that I've lived in a community with access to fresh, nutritious food and made a choice to eat junk every day. I live in the Midwest. Vegetables, grains, and livestock are grown all around me. My entire state is a farmer's market in the summer! It is also ironic (and a little sad) that my husband provided me with a comfortable household income since day one of our marriage, and we still lived paycheck to paycheck.

I am not a physician, but I have self-diagnosed the condition I suffered from for many years. The common term is the Ostrich Syndrome. It is defined as denying or refusing to acknowledge something that is blatantly obvious as if "your head is in the sand." Like the ostrich, I hid from the truth all around me because of fear and ignorance. It put pounds on my body and added weight to my debt.

Let's pluck some of these ostrich feathers and see what lurks underneath:

1. **"Go ahead and buy it. Just put it on the credit card and pay it off later."** The Ostrich Fear: If my family doesn't have the best house, electronics, clothes, cars, vacations, and so on, they will be mocked or treated differently. I will look like a bad parent and a bad spouse.

2. **"Go ahead and it eat. My day has been so hectic, and I deserve a quick treat. I'll start the diet when things calm down a little bit."** The Ostrich Fear: Facing my obesity is too hard. I know I'll starve and be miserable. A diet today is a terrible idea. A diet tomorrow is a good idea, and a diet next week is an even better idea.

3. **"No need to open that bank statement. It will just be depressing."** The Ostrich Fear: I hate looking at these numbers. They just prove that I'm facing a mess that I can't fix.

4. **"No need to get on a scale. No need to find out how many calories I'm eating every day. It will just be depressing."** The Ostrich Fear (which is, interestingly enough, the same as above): I hate

looking at these numbers. They just prove that I'm facing a mess that I can't fix.

5. **"Eat, drink, and be merry because trying to make a change is pointless. It's too late, and I've made too many mistakes."** The Ostrich Fear: God may be big, but my problems are bigger.

If you are reading this and know (to the exact dollar) the amount of money in your checking account, get ready for some good news. If you pay off your credit cards every month (or don't use credit cards at all), you have a weight-loss advantage that will be an amazing thing to behold. If you always spend less than you make (and invest the rest), you understand that paying attention to the "little" things today can make big things happen for you in the future.

To all of those Dave Ramsey fans out there, it's time to put those money skills to work on your diet plan. In this book you will learn that weight loss is as straight forward as:

1. **Knowing the calories you consume and how many calories are within your healthy, daily budget.** At any point during the day, you should know your current balance. When your account is at zero, stop eating or go for a long walk.

2. **Avoiding calorie debt.** This is a math equation. Output (calories burned) should always be greater than input (calories consumed).

3. **Understanding that even a small amount of weight loss each week will pay big returns in the future.** Think compounding interest!

If you are reading this and your idea of financial planning is playing the lottery (thank you for the joke, Jeff Foxworthy), welcome home. You and I possibly fell out of the same ostrich nest. Weight loss for us is more difficult because we have fear in more than one area of our lives. We alternate between dreaming and hiding. On a good day (such as payday) we dream that our problems will magically melt away...preferably with very little effort on our part. On a bad day (such as when we start getting collection calls or can't fit into our jeans anymore) we hide our heads and refuse to face the truth.

I am pleased to tell you, my fellow birdbrain, that we are not a lost cause. Our steps toward lowering our weight and raising our credit scores are different from those diversified investors above. The road will be steep, but reaching our destination will be just as sweet. It starts by:

1. **Realizing that God wants you to move forward with your hand in His and your eyes open.** If your spouse suddenly gets a big raise at work, you will still live paycheck to paycheck if you don't understand where your money is being spent. If your spouse is losing weight, you won't be one pound lighter if you don't know how many calories you are eating. God asks each one of us to walk in the light of His truth, not in the blind "get fixed quick" schemes of the world. Pull your head out and wipe the sand from your eyes. You will no longer live life like an ostrich.

2. **Understanding that the real number to focus on is time.** Most Americans would be happy with a bigger bank account and a smaller waistline. Those are the digits that get our attention, but it must start with a commitment of our time. Balancing your checking account, making a budget, and calculating your daily calories will take minutes out of your day.

For me it meant watching less television. I had to make room in my schedule to get healthy.

3. **Taking hope from your achievements.** This is perhaps the best news of all. When you have success living within a budget, *a calorie budget or a financial budget*, your courage to tackle new challenges grows. You will have the patience to endure slow and steady progress and a renewed faith in what the Lord can accomplished through you.

"He that is faithful in that which is least is faithful also in much."[1] Your "least" on the Skinny Budget Diet might be ordering chicken soup instead of french fries. Your "least" might be putting away your credit cards and waiting until you can pay cash. I can tell you *as one former ostrich to another* that your "least" will feel like "much" when God blesses your work and faithfulness. Let's get started!

Chapter One

WASTING TIME ON A GROWING WAIST

I WROTE THIS BOOK for you. And throughout these chapters you and I are going to get very close. There will be no such thing as TMI. I am happy to provide "too much information" on every page of this book if it will give you your life back. Want to hear about the roller coasters I couldn't fit into or the lawn chairs I broke when I weighed three hundred pounds? You got it. I'll even give you the blow-by-blow of how I shaved my legs every day without the ability to see my feet.

It may not be pretty stuff, but I think it is important for you to understand that there is no such thing as "too broken" or "too far gone." And while I'm not a fan of beating myself up over bad choices, you can learn from my twenty years of mistakes. I wasted thousands of dollars trying to buy my way out of obesity. It left me with a heavier body, heavier debt, and some heavy lies in my head: 'I really shouldn't eat the rest of these cookies. Oh, go ahead. You are so fat...what's a few more pounds? But what if I can't find clothes that fit anymore? This little plate of cookies won't make any difference. You work hard. You deserve a treat."

I wish I could claim that underlying mental scars or repressed abuse led to my constant cycle of overeating and guilt. It didn't. I could tell you that I was obese because of past pregnancies and post-baby weight. My youngest son weighed more than twelve pounds at birth. *Twelve pounds!* But that wasn't the reason for my obesity.

I ate when I was happy—to celebrate friends and family, to reward myself after a stressful day of work, even to enjoy my favorite TV shows. I ate because food tasted good. When I left my mom's healthy table and went to college, I gained my "freshman fifteen" and kept on going. I can't blame my obesity on a thyroid problem or even a slow metabolism. I ate myself to morbid obesity through daily, unhealthy choices—each seeming so small and insignificant at the time.

There are as many reasons for overeating as flavors at Baskin-Robbins. You may have a story that is similar to mine, or your story may be filled with true sadness. I understand that food can be an anesthesia to make the world seem less painful or a weapon to keep the world a safe distance away.

It is not my intention to minimize the underlying causes of obesity. We'll get into some of these reasons in more detail as we work through this book. At the moment simply understand that your reasons for overeating can no longer be used as excuses to stay obese. Excuses (even excuses that seem valid) won't make you one pound lighter. They serve no purpose for good.

Two Decades of Weight-Loss "Practice"

"Honey, you have such a pretty face. Have you tried losing weight?" I'm generally not a violent person, but questions like that made me see red. If I could have lifted my foot above my waist, I would have kicked these well-meaning, skinny people in the gut...or the ribs...or whatever thin people have around their waists in the place of fat. Have I *tried* losing weight? You can't be serious!

I had more failed weight-loss plans in my past than candy wrappers on the bottom of my purse. Each one had a price tag. At the time did I understand the science of losing weight? You bet. I was an obese woman living in the United States. As a group we are probably more informed about calories and exercise than the general public. Ironic, isn't it? I've spent hours watching people "sweat to the oldies" and sculpt "buns of steel." I have vivid memories of spreading cream cheese on a bagel while watching Tony Horton sell his latest exercise plan.

I think the biggest myth going is that obese Americans don't understand how they became overweight and have no idea how to lose it. Here is one lie that I always told myself: "I'm so confused. I don't know whether to count calories, carbs, or fat." That excuse was a great way to start a heated debate in any crowd and kill my dieting plans before lunch.

The results of all these failed diet attempts were damaging—not only physically but also spiritually. I began to truly believe that:

1. Losing weight the "old fashioned way" with diet and exercise is too hard and takes too long.

2. People who lose weight and keep it off obviously have more willpower than I do. "Face it, Linda. There must be something wrong your character. You are just too weak to lose weight."

3. Maybe it is God's plan for me to be this big. After all, He created each one of us to be unique and different. I'm *supposed* to be three hundred pounds.

Most of us are obese because we eat more food than our bodies can burn, and we've been doing it for years. Mystery solved! What's not as easy to understand is the role that the brain plays in this behavior. I've tried to honestly examine the choices I made at three hundred pounds, and the constant dialogue that ran through my brain. I think some of my daily thoughts about food may sound familiar to you. And so I present...

A DAY IN THE LIFE OF A CHRONIC DIETER		
Time	Thoughts in My Head	What I Ate
6:30 a.m.	Wake up the kids. Make their breakfast and pack their lunches. No time for breakfast right now. And besides, today you start the diet.	Nothing
6:50 a.m.	I hate my clothes. Time to pull out the black skirt...again. Should I wear a higher heel? No, too painful. Stick with flats. Jewelry? What's the point?	
7:45 a.m.	I'm starving. Grab something for breakfast on the way to work.	Two bacon, egg, and cheese biscuits from McDonald's (and a Diet Coke to keep my calories down)
10:00 a.m.	What should I have for lunch?	
10:30 a.m.	What sounds good for lunch?	
11:00 a.m.	Should I invite Pam out to lunch? Probably not. She will order something healthy liked grilled fish, and you'll look like a fat pig.	
11:30 a.m.	Drive to Panera Bread now or you'll miss the beginning of your TV show.	
12:00 p.m.	Lunch. Remember, be healthy. Skip the potato chips and get an apple instead.	One Panera Italian combo sandwich, an apple, and a frozen mocha to drink
1:30 p.m.	I need a nap.	

A DAY IN THE LIFE OF A CHRONIC DIETER		
Time	**Thoughts in My Head**	**What I Ate**
2:00 pm.	Appointment upstairs. Better take the elevator. You'll be huffing and wheezing during the first five minutes of the meeting if you take the stairs.	
3:00 p.m.	I really need a nap.	
3:30 p.m.	I better make an ice cream run or I'm going to fall asleep at my desk. Hey, bring back ice cream for the whole office. It will be like a party!	One medium chocolate dipped strawberry Blizzard from Dairy Queen
4:30 a.m.	Oh…man! I forgot to defrost something for dinner. Maybe I can just pick up some pizza on the way home from work. Make a big salad to go with it. Without the ranch dressing, it will be healthy.	One-third of a large Meat Lover's pan pizza from Pizza Hut and a salad with cheese, croutons and a low-fat Italian dressing
9:00 p.m.	The boys are finally in bed, and you have a couple hours of peace with that handsome man of yours. Hey, the cute pie shop uptown doesn't close until 10:00 p.m. Make a pie run but no whipped cream. Watching those calories!	One slice of Toll House pie
10:30 p.m.	Don't take off your clothes until the lights are out. ALL of the lights. I wish I were skinny. Monday. Start the new diet on Monday.	Total calories consumed: 5,000+

Looking at my "Day in the Life of" menu, I don't know whether to laugh or cry. It is a true account of the crazy, internal battles of an obese woman. Being this honest may not be easy for you, but here is what I learned by writing down my daily menu:

1. I had no idea at the time how many calories I was eating. If you quizzed me as I was brushing my teeth before bed, I would have guessed that I'd eaten about three thousand calories, not a button-popping five-thousand-plus in just one day. I'd skipped the Coke, potato chips, ranch dressing, and whipped cream. That's healthy, right?

2. Most of my food was coming from restaurants and not grocery stores. This is an important thing to realize...both in regard to maintaining a healthy weight and a healthy wallet. More on this later.

3. I often ate while doing other things such as driving, working, and watching television.

4. Frustration about dieting and weight loss was often my first thought of the day and the last thing in my head before falling asleep. So many precious hours that I gave away to my obesity.

5. My size was changing my life: the clothes I wore, the people I ate with, and the intimacy I had with my husband.

As I was starting diet number forty-seven (or maybe it was diet number forty-nine), I caught an interview with NBC weatherman Al Roker in which he talked about his gastric bypass surgery. It was a fascinating idea to me. You just make your stomach smaller and force yourself to eat less food. If you screw up, you throw up. Genius!

I was now a woman on a mission, searching the web and reading every magazine article I could find with details on the procedure. The before and after pictures for celebrities such as Carnie Wilson, Roseanne Barr, and Al Roker were amazing. They had lost hundreds of pounds in a short amount of time. Gastric bypass surgery was going to be my answer, my quick escape from morbid obesity.

MY GASTRIC BYPASS OBSESSION

I contacted a surgical weight-loss center in 2002 and began the long, pre-surgical process that included a consultation with a psychologist, an exam with my local doctor, and blood work. My primary physician went over the risks for gastric bypass surgery in great detail, and I'm sure that I smiled and nodded back when she told me that:

1. The procedure has a death rate that some doctors estimate to be as high as one in one hundred. What went through my head: "Those are still pretty good odds, right?"

2. The surgery can lead to vitamin and mineral deficiencies requiring daily supplements and B_{12} shots at least once a week. My thoughts: "Maybe Flintstone vitamins will come out with B_{12} in a gummy fruit. That would be cool."

3. There is a syndrome called dumping where your food can move too quickly through the small intestine causing nausea, diarrhea, and vomiting. Inside my head: "Did she just say something about a dump? What?"

There was a big disconnect between the information given to me by my doctor and what I was focused on. When you believe that gastric bypass is your only ticket out of morbid obesity, the risks don't matter. I was willing to live with almost anything to be thin…especially if the solution didn't require a lot of willpower on my part.

From all of my research I knew that qualifying for gastric bypass surgery wasn't going to be easy. I had to show my insurance company that I was *unhealthy* enough to need the procedure but *healthy* enough to live through the surgery. My weight wasn't a problem. With a BMI (body mass index) between 47 and 48, I met that requirement. A healthy BMI range is between 18.5 and 24.9. I also had to show a history of failed dieting attempts. That was an easy requirement after two decades of being obese.

I was happy (practically giddy) the day I mailed my huge stack of forms back to the surgical weight-loss center. Clearance from my doctor and psychologist? Check. Blood work proving that I didn't have thyroid issues? Check. The name and policy number for my insurance company? Check. I was cleared to have the surgery and ready for takeoff.

Unfortunately my insurance company didn't agree. My calls to the surgical weight-loss center became more frequent as the weeks went by. A very patient lady in the admissions department gave me updates about her discussions with my insurance company. Even with gallbladder disease, occasional chest pains, and a scale at three hundred pounds, my insurance company said I didn't have enough risk factors to justify the surgery. I wasn't diabetic—yet. I didn't have high blood pressure or breathing problems—yet. Basically I was too healthy.

From Little Control to Out of Control

The day I received the final no from my insurance company is one I will never forget. I was crushed. I believed my insurance company had just sentenced me to a lifetime of morbid obesity. I was so angry inside I gave up on the idea of ever trying to diet or exercise. If I needed to be "sick" to qualify for the surgery, fine.

Diabetes is common in my family, so I'll just keep eating. Maybe my insurance company will pay for the procedure if I weigh three hundred fifty pounds. And I'm sure I will get the green light if I weigh four hundred pounds.

Looking back, my daily plan to add another hundred pounds was nearly flawless. It could have been called a personal weight-gain plan. I ignored food labels, lived in the drive-through lane, and ate whatever was put in front of me. I even stopped going to the doctor so that I could skip that awkward "let's get your weight" moment. I went three years without a yearly exam or checkup of any kind.

There are very few "before" pictures of me during this time. I remember sitting in my car and going through stacks of developed pictures. Before letting anyone else see the pictures, I would throw away any photos showing my body (especially from the side). When my boys look back at their childhood photo albums, they are going to wonder if their mother ran off with the circus during this period of their lives. My kids loved disposable cameras and knew that they could take pictures of their dad, the dog, even our half-dead cat, but never, *never* take a picture of mom.

I was hiding from my appearance, and I honestly have no idea how much I weighed at my heaviest. I do know that I didn't fit in airplane seats, roller-coaster seats, theater seats, or even the seats at some of my favorite restaurants. How is that for irony? I was wearing a size 4X, and buying clothes was a horrendous experience.

There are a few things in the world that I've always found impossible: folding a fitted sheet, safely clipping my cat's claws, and finding size 26 clothes that made me "look skinny." At three hundred pounds, shopping for jeans was an aerobic activity that often left me sweating. I'd walk into the dressing room, turn away from the mirror, and do the dance.

Do you know the one? You start by jumping up and down to get the denim around your lumpy parts. Follow that up by lying flat on the ground to get the jeans buttoned. If you are successful with the first two steps, it's time for the final challenge. You must get back on your feet without popping a button or ripping out the seams in your seat.

It was generally in these dignified moments that I asked myself, "When did I get this large? What am I going to do when even the plus size clothes are too small? How did I let myself get this out of control?"

I enjoy living in a small town, but the closest mall is more than one hour away. I remember being so relieved when a local clothing store expanded their sizes beyond a 3X. It can be terrifying when your body is too large to wear *anything* in the store. Forget about dressing fashionably, I was just worried about dressing at all.

WHEN MY BOTTOM HIT BOTTOM

The stages of obesity are strangely similar to the stages of grief. If you've struggled with your weight for a long time, you may see yourself in one of the phases below. Because I'm such an over-achiever, I had to hit all five stages before my bottom hit bottom. It was a twenty-year spiral down.

1. **Denial:** "I'm not obese. I just have a lot of curves. This can't be happening...not to me. Gaining a few extra pounds is simply a part of getting older, right? I don't have the metabolism I had in high school, but it's not like I have a serious problem."

2. **Anger:** "It's not fair. If my spouse (children, friends, coworkers, and so on) didn't sit around eating so many high-calorie foods, I wouldn't have this problem. How could anyone lose weight with this many temptations? They are to blame." Once we are in the second stage, we recognize that denial cannot continue.

3. **Bargaining:** "I know I have a problem. I'm going to lose the weight but not today. My schedule is just too hectic, and I'm too stressed out. I'll start the diet on Monday." In this stage we want more time before confronting the tough work we see ahead of us.

4. **Depression:** "Why even bother to try anymore? What is the point of starting another diet? This isn't going to work anyway. I might as well eat whatever I feel like. I'm always going to be fat." This was the stage for me where I gave up on weight loss and exercise completely. I stopped going to the doctor so I didn't have to get on the scale and I started making fat jokes at my own expense to cover my pain.

5. **Acceptance:** This is the hour, the minute, the second when you finally hit bottom. If you've ever fought an addiction and won, acceptance is a moment in time you will never forget. Mine was a Saturday morning in March 2007 at about 7:30 a.m. Oh yes, I can be that specific.

I think the world has a misconception about acceptance. We imagine people standing up, dusting off their hands, and working to fix their problems. There is actually more to it than that. Acceptance is when you are willing to put your trust in something beyond yourself. It is an attitude that "I will do whatever it takes, no matter how hard, because I can't live like this anymore. I will no longer value pride over health. I need help, and I'm not going to be afraid to ask for it."

For the first fifteen years of my obesity I bounced from anger (when a weight-loss plan didn't work) back to bargaining (before I started the next diet). After being told no to gastric bypass surgery by my insurance company, I finally slid into the depression stage. I gave up on weight loss and ate whatever was in front of me.

When I travel and speak with groups, I get these questions more than any other: What happened in 2007? Why did you lose the weight? That question makes me sweat! For more than a year I gave the safe, comfortable answer that I wanted to be healthier and set a good example for my children. And while that is true, it wasn't a part of my "bottom hitting bottom" moment.

I'm going to be honest here because I believe it is important for other married people to understand that they aren't alone. One weekend in March of 2007 it became clear to me that the awesome man I married couldn't pretend to find me attractive anymore. Our intimacy was precious to me, and we were losing it. I was daring him to find me attractive at two hundred pounds, two hundred fifty pounds...OK, how about three hundred pounds? It was like my weight was a third person lying in our bed between us. I saw a day coming when we would live together "just as friends," and it broke my heart.

I have to stop for a moment and tell you a little bit about my husband. When we said our marriage vows in 1992, the man was *serious*. I never worried for one minute that he would cheat on me or want a divorce. Every day he told me he loved me. It was just a problem that there seemed to be a lot more of me to love every day.

I don't believe that wives should torture themselves trying to look like models. Let's be honest. Even a supermodel doesn't really look like a supermodel when you take away the hour of expert makeup and the magic of Photoshop. I do think we owe it to our spouses, however, to take care of ourselves. At three hundred pounds I stopped getting haircuts, considered makeup a waste of time, and avoided mirrors like the plague. Men are visual. God created them that way, and I can only imagine how tired my husband must have been seeing me in baggy sweatpants every day.

I think my "bottom smacking" moment went back to those marriage vows we had said to each other fifteen years earlier. My husband promised to love me in sickness and in health, but I was *choosing* sickness over health. It wasn't fair to him. My out-of-control eating habits and lack of exercise were hurting my marriage and slowly killing me. I was ready to lose weight like a grown-up.

Does this mean that I lost 155 pounds for my husband? No. I didn't lose the weight for him. I lost the weight for us. I think if my only motivation had been to make my husband happy, my diet wouldn't have lasted a week. This is at the core of why we can't nag, badger, or beg our spouses to be healthier. A guilt trip or mean comments from my husband would have sent me to the nearest buffet line with a battle cry of, "You think I'm fat? I'll show you fat!"

Your parents may be worried sick about your growing size. Your spouse may be secretly throwing away your snacks. Your kids may dream of having a parent who is active and involved. That alone won't be enough. A healthier you is a gift to those who love you, but it is a gift that must be given of your own free will. Has your bottom touched bottom?

FROM WILLPOWER TO "THY WILL" POWER

"I tell you the truth, if you have faith as small as a mustard seed, you can say to this mountain, 'Move from here to there' and it will move. Nothing will be impossible for you."[1]

I did a little bit of research about the mustard seed. It is generally about three millimeters in diameter and is one of the smallest seeds on the planet. What I found interesting is that the tiny mustard seed can grow to be one of the largest plants in the garden. But in March of 2007 all I knew about mustard was that it tasted great on a hot dog.

Looking back, the mustard seed really was the perfect symbol for where I was at in my head. Because of so many past diet failures I had almost no faith that I would ever lose weight. I had almost no faith that God would listen to my prayers. I had almost no faith that He could give me the strength to try again…almost.

It turns out that the three millimeters of faith that I had in my heart was enough. Actually it was more than enough.

To say that I probably didn't look my best on that day in March of 2007 would be an understatement. I want you to give you clear picture of my "before" photo—no touch-ups. It was early on a Saturday morning, so you have to picture an obese woman with her hair standing straight up, not a lot of clothes on, and teeth that probably needed to be brushed. My eyes were practically swollen shut from my tears, and an occasional snot-bubble is not outside the realm of possibility. I looked *rough*. God didn't care.

He listened to me make an ugly, honest confession. I had allowed food to be my god. It had become my comforter and my crutch. And if you've struggled with your weight or with *any* addiction, you know that it can be an angry and unforgiving god. The very day I cried out and prayed for help, God (with the big, capital G) gave me a no-thank-you muscle I never had before.

Here is the best way I can describe it. When an obese person sees something delicious on a plate, the "must have it" meter is off the charts. A piece of warm apple pie with vanilla ice cream would be an eighteen for me on a scale of one to ten. It was impossible to resist. On the Saturday I asked God to carry me, my "must have it" meter for the foods I loved was immediately dialed down. The food still looked delicious, but I didn't feel as if I would die if I simply said, "No, thank you."

That feeling of strength has never left me. It gave my soul the courage to try again even after two decades of failure. It gave my brain the opportunity to put the science of weight loss into action. God took my faith (the size of a mustard seed) and moved a mountain; a 155-pound mountain of fat to be exact.

If you can take away just one thing from my story, I hope it is this. God is still in the miracle business. I learned in a very real way that God has plans for us. Plans to prosper us and not to harm us. Plans to give us hope and a future.[2] The Father who created you and can count every hair on your head is not a deadbeat dad.

We're going to talk about the role that faith and support can play for you, but our first hour class is science. Don't worry. You won't need a periodic table of the elements or a Bunsen burner. In the next chapter I want to give you some basic facts about how our bodies work, use calories, and store fuel. There is a measurement tool called the body mass index and my own creation called a brain mass index. Both can be eye opening.

House Call With Rita Hancock, MD

Question: I have a long list of diets in my past. Many of them were all about restrictions and what foods I could and couldn't eat. Do you ever wonder what God thinks about our constant dieting?

Dr. Hancock: I think it breaks God's heart to see us suffer with the consequences of obesity, but I also think it breaks His heart to see us chronically diet and fail. Our failures just compound the feelings of helplessness and hopelessness that lead to emotional eating. Plus, dieting fuels our obsession with food. It makes us want the food we think we shouldn't eat even more. It's a vicious, self-defeating cycle.

Because each of us is so different (for example, for some of us restricting dieting backfires), I don't believe God would advocate a single, one-size-fits-all diet for all Christians. No doubt God would give each of us an individualized diet if we lived in an ideal world where we could hear His instructions clearly.

Unfortunately we don't live in an ideal world. Being that we're all unique, individual creations, and being that we're all imperfect, God gave us only *general* guidelines to follow in Scripture. Let's look at those general guidelines here:

1. You shouldn't be gluttonous (Prov. 23:2, 20–21).

2. You shouldn't worry about or think too much about what you will eat (Matt. 6:25).

3. You can eat any type of food (Mark 7:15–19).

4. You should eat to the glory of God (1 Cor. 10:31).

Let's take a minute to talk about each of these scriptures specifically. First, think about the meaning of gluttony. Generally most would agree that it means, "overeating." But how much is too much? Are you gluttonous if you eat twenty cookies? Most would say yes. How about if you eat two cookies? And can you be gluttonous in ways other than eating? The exact definition of gluttony can be hard to pin down, if you ask me.

Second, do you worry too much about food and eating? A long time ago I was in bondage to food. I was either on a diet or off a diet, as if I was on a dieting roller coaster. My first thought in the morning was either, "Feed me!" or "I hope I don't overeat today," depending on which part of the roller coaster I was on.

I most definitely thought about food more than I thought about God. In fact, my obsessive thoughts about food actually drove a wedge between God and me. That's why I think it was bondage.

Eventually, by the grace of God and using methods I discuss further in *The Eden Diet*, I was able to break free from this bondage and reestablish the right pecking order. Jesus was Lord over me, and I was lord over the food.

Third, Scripture says you can eat any type of food. Notice that God didn't say carrot sticks are morally superior to cheesecake. At the same rate Paul pointed out that just because something is allowable, it isn't necessarily advisable. People with fat-clogged arteries ought to avoid eating more than a few bites of cheesecake, lest they have heart attacks and die. The point is, you must use common sense and eat potentially unhealthy food in small amounts, especially if you're trying to lose weight or if you have unique medical needs that require you to follow a strict diet.

Fourth, you should eat with an attitude of thankfulness and reverence to God. Eating with the proper attitude, that is, without anxiety and guilt, leads to greater satisfaction with the eating experience so that less food equals more joy.

Rita Hancock, MD, is a Christian physician with Ivy League nutrition training and studies of obese psychology. She draws upon her faith and her personal success overcoming childhood-onset obesity to help those in bondage to food, eating, and dieting. To learn more about Dr. Hancock's work or purchase The Eden Diet *or other resources developed by Dr. Hancock, visit her website at www.theedendiet.com.*

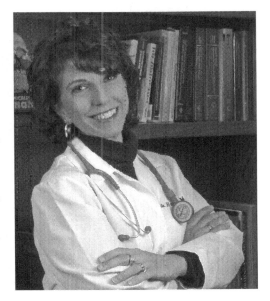

Chapter Two

SEPARATING THE FACTS
FROM FAT FICTION

L ET'S START THIS chapter with some controversy. It is my opinion that you can be perfectly healthy and still be classified as overweight. Your negative label may not come from family or friends but from your BMI. This calculation takes your height and weight and puts you into one of four categories: underweight, normal, overweight, or obese.

The purpose of the BMI is to provide a reliable indicator of body fatness and screen for weight categories that may lead to health problems. You can calculate your BMI for free at www.cdc.gov/healthyweight.

The BMI guidelines are wonderful tools, but don't let them be the final word about your weight. Some people have greater energy, strength, and endurance when they carry a few extra pounds. I'm starting to worry at this point that the BMI police will break down my door and haul me away. But we're going to continue and not be afraid!

Call it anecdotal evidence, but I remember the farmers I grew up around in Northern Missouri. Many of these individuals (men and women) were not what you would call petite flowers. And while they wouldn't be classified on the BMI scale as obese, they would have been considered overweight and advised by the Centers for Disease Control and Prevention that even a small weight loss of 10 percent may lower their risk for disease.[1]

It's important to consider, however, what the BMI scales don't take into account. They are designed to be a diagnostic tool but can't determine an individual's percentage of body fat or overall state of health. My farming neighbors in Missouri lifted and carried everything from bags of seed to baby calves and probably walked ten miles a day. These were individuals who did most of their cardiovascular work wearing a pair of cowboy boots.

So what does that mean to you? If your occupation or lifestyle keeps you active (and you've got the muscle tone to prove it), don't rely on the body mass index alone to determine if you need to lose some weight. Talk to your doctor and get a second opinion about your size, waist circumference, and percentage of body fat. It's time for a physical!

If you don't have high blood pressure, high LDL cholesterol, low HDL cholesterol, high levels of triglycerides, or type 2 diabetes, your current weight may be considered healthy even if it's above the "normal" BMI range. Your doctor is going to be your best source of information even beyond the numbers. He or she should ask for your medical history and know if your family is predisposed to cancer, heart disease, strokes, and the like.

THE BEER BELLY POLKA TEST

By the end of my freshman year at University of Missouri I thought I had men figured out. My education about the males on this planet started during the infamous "sixth grade talk" and continued unceasingly through my first year in college. My fellow classmates on the subject of men were generally the other confused young ladies in my dorm. My lessons always started with this question: Why do guys *do* that?

I was nineteen years old that spring in 1987 and confident that I finally had an A in Men 101. Nothing a man could do would surprise me anymore. All of my arrogance died one day during finals week when I found an open seat in the library, looked up, and saw the T-shirt on the young man seated across from me.

The shirt read, "Beer belly under construction." And just in case that wasn't clear enough, a bright orange arrow pointed to his personal belly "blueprint." It was a construction project that had to be close to completion. This guy had clearly attended more than a few parties during his college career and probably had a seat of honor right next to the keg.

I gave up that day. I would never completely understand men, and I stopped trying. My only hope was that this type of humorous T-shirt wouldn't become fashionable for women. I was about thirty pounds overweight after my freshman year and too sensitive to make jokes at my own expense. Looking back, I had nothing to be afraid of. Most females would rather die than wear a T-shirt that reads, "I think my ankles were stolen. I haven't seen them since 1986."

Whether you try to hide your stomach under loose-fitting clothes or carry it under a T-shirt with pride, it can't be ignored when we talk about weight loss. It's not healthy for anyone to dance the beer belly polka. In the past physicians simply used a scale to determine if a patient was at a healthy weight. Belly fat on men and women who fell within normal weight ranges was largely ignored. If the average Joe was five feet ten inches tall and weighed 173 pounds, his overall size would have been considered healthy by his doctor. What's a bulging belly between friends? Unfortunately for Joe physicians now know that skinny arms and legs may not keep Joe from an early grave.

We've been told for years that excess body fat increases our risk for heart disease, strokes, and diabetes. Research published in the *New England Journal of Medicine* suggests that the distribution of our fat can be just as important as our BMI when determining the risk of an early death.[2] This research comes from a European study that followed nearly 360,000 people for ten years, making it one of the largest, longest studies on belly fat.

The 2008 report found that people with a higher percentage of belly fat had nearly twice the risk of dying prematurely as people with a smaller percentage of belly fat. The death risk increased with waist circumference whether the participants were overweight or not. So how can we determine if our passive pooch has become a more problematic paunch?

Let's forget about our bathroom scales for a moment and pull out a tape measure. For most men the risk factors for disease increase with a waist size greater than 40 inches. The same is true for women when their waist sizes are greater than 34.6 inches. Dig a tape measure out of your sewing kit (or the junk drawer in my case) and we'll get started.

1. Place a tape measure around your bare abdomen just above your hipbone.

2. Pull until it fits snugly around you but doesn't push into your skin. Make sure the tape measure is level all the way around and lying flat against your body.

3. Exhale and measure your waist. Don't cheat and suck in your gut. Save that trick for impressing members of the opposite sex. We need an accurate measurement today.

While you have the tape measure out, you will also want to measure the circumference of your hips. Place the tape measure around the largest part of your hips (generally at the widest part of the buttocks). Divide your waist size by your hip size. For men a ratio of .90 or less is considered ideal. For women a ratio of .80 or less is our goal. (You have finally found a place, ladies, where wider hips are good news!)

Even without the power of a tape measure, most of us can use a mirror to determine if we have a pear-shaped body or an apple-shaped body. Research shows that "pear people" tend to have fewer diseases and live longer. This is one situation where an apple a day won't keep the doctor away.

If seeing your individual waist to hip ratio was depressing, don't despair! We have some work to do, but there is hope for anyone with too much apple in his shadow.

HEARTY AND HEALTHY VS. SKINNY AND SICK

In addition to the opinion of your doctor and the notches on your belt, there are daily activities that can provide you with valuable health information about your current size and level of endurance. I recently had an opportunity to witness an impromptu fitness test firsthand. And yes, I was eavesdropping.

In small doses I think it can be fun to watch teenagers gossip, gawk, gesture, and giggle. I stayed behind a young pack of students leaving a school event and matched their pace through several parking lots and up a hill. My car was about four hundred yards away, and we all seemed to be walking in the same direction.

After a few minutes I stopped listening to the group's words and began listening to the group's breathing. Several were now panting between sentences, and not the "love panting" you remember as a teenager. I'm talking about panting for air.

No offense to anyone else who cheered for the 1980 US hockey team, but these young people sounded more like their parents. Was I hearing forty-three-year-old lungs or seventeen-year-old lungs at work? I spent the remainder of my hike to the car trying to figure it out.

- **How steep was this hill we were climbing?** I wouldn't want to scale it with a piano on my back, but by Ozark Mountain standards, the hill wasn't that intimidating.

- **Were these students at a healthy weight?** I know from experience that packing extra pounds can make even the smallest hill feel like Mount Everest. This group, however, wasn't overweight. Two of the young ladies were close to my height and probably fifteen pounds lighter.

- **Was this hill changing my breathing?** Silently trailing a group of socializing teenagers wasn't a fair comparison. I needed to use my voice, and that gave me two options. I could talk to myself and look mentally unbalanced, or I could sing to myself and simply appear eccentric. I chose eccentric and quietly sang my ABCs. It wasn't exactly *American Idol* material, but I didn't forget the lyrics. I made it to the letter V before I needed a breath to stay comfortable.

My unplanned and unscientific research was done. Unless these students were all suffering with asthma, bronchitis, or emphysema, they weren't as "in shape" as they should have been. I was seeing the skinny sick in action…or as much action as their lungs could probably stand. I knew a secret about these teenagers that perhaps their parents and doctors didn't even realize.

As long as "Jessica" still fits in her size 5 jeans, will mom and dad automatically assume that they have a healthy daughter? As long as "Aaron" has flat abs and the right number on the scale, will his doctor guess that the young man has the endurance of someone twenty years older? It's a "sick secret" that even the skinny themselves may not be aware of.

Researchers are finding that being skinny isn't necessarily the same thing as being healthy. In fact, some reports show that maintaining a normal weight may not save us from the disease risks of a sedentary lifestyle. We'll talk more about how to start moving in a later chapter. There is some good news for all the fitness lovers out there who can't seem to lose the last twenty-five pounds.

So let's make this personal. Do you consider yourself active? I've discovered something humorous about this question. It's a lot like asking a group of parents if their preschooler has above average intelligence. Nearly everyone will answer yes. I don't think it is a case of flagrant fibbing. We confuse busyness with fitness. We confuse hectic schedules and a stressful work environment with being active. We confuse sweating from the heat with sweating from exercise. Not everything that puts your deodorant to the test is created equal.

The American Council on Exercise has a quick and inexpensive way to find your general fitness level. I researched several at-home options, and I like this one because it doesn't require the purchase of a treadmill or extra equipment. All you need is a flat surface, a pair of tennis shoes, and a watch with a second hand. Get the green light from your doctor before you take the test, and let's see what you can do.

THE ONE-MILE WALKING TEST

Your goal is to walk one mile as quickly as possible and record your time. It could change your results if you run this test on a hilly surface (and leave you depressed with the results), so find a flat sidewalk, road, or track. Four laps is one mile on a standard track at your local high school. And for all the overachievers in the crowd, jogging instead of walking is fine if you are feeling energetic. These are the age-adjusted standards according to the American Council on Exercise.[3]

1. **Men age twenty to twenty-nine:** An excellent time is under eleven minutes and fifty-four seconds (11:54), average is under thirteen minutes and forty-two seconds (13:42), and poor is classified as fourteen minutes and thirty seconds (14:30) or longer.

2. **Men age thirty to thirty-nine:** Excellent is under 12:24, average is under 14:12, and poor is 15:00 or longer.

3. **Men age forty to forty-nine:** Excellent is under 12:54, average is under 14:42, and poor is 15:30 or longer.

4. **Men age fifty to fifty-nine:** Excellent is under 13:24, average is under 15:12, and poor is 16:30 or longer.

5. **Men age sixty to sixty-nine:** Excellent is under 14:06, average is under 16:18, and poor is 17:18 or longer.

6. **Men age seventy or older:** Excellent is under 15:06, average is under 18:48, and poor is 20:18 or longer.

The standards are a little different for the ladies:

7. **Women age of twenty to twenty-nine:** An excellent time is under thirteen minutes and twelve seconds (13:12), average is under fifteen minutes and six seconds (15:06), and poor is classified as sixteen minutes and thirteen seconds (16:30) or longer.

8. **Women age thirty to thirty-nine:** Excellent is under 13:42, average is under 15:36, and poor is 17:00 or longer.

9. **Women age forty to forty-nine:** Excellent is under 14:12, average is under 16:06, and poor is 17:30 or longer.

10. **Women age fifty to fifty-nine:** Excellent is under 14:42, average is under 17:00, and poor is 18:06 or longer.

11. **Women age sixty to sixty-nine:** Excellent is under 15:06, average is under 17:30, and poor is 19:12 or longer.

12. **Women age seventy or older:** Excellent is under 18:18, average is under 21:48, and poor is 24:06 or longer.

Before you lace up your sneakers and hit the pavement, I have one final reminder. Don't let the results of this test leave you feeling hopeless. At age thirty-nine and with a weight of three-hundred-plus pounds, my one-mile walking time would have been somewhere between twenty minutes and the moment when Jesus returns. I was the definition of "out of shape." Over the last few years I've made steady progress. The Lord built each one of us with the ability to improve our strength and endurance at any age. I am literally walking proof that we are fearfully and wonderfully made.[4]

How Heavy Is Your Head? The Brain Test

I would now like to introduce you to another BMI scale that I feel is just as important as the body mass index. Let's call it the brain mass index. And no, we're not going to blame our weight struggles on an oversized cranium.

I want you to take a moment and calculate how many minutes on average you spend every day feeling unhappy about your current size and guilty about the food you eat. It is a powerful way to determine if you are piloting your own plate or if your plate is piloting you.

Don't simply say to yourself, "Yeah, I probably focus on food a lot." You need to write the final number down and look at it . . . *really* look at it. This is important, and it is for your eyes only. Grab a calculator or write your math in the margin. No one will slap your hand with a ruler.

Average number of minutes I spend thinking about my weight every day   _____

Average number of minutes I spend thinking about my food   _____

Average number of minutes every day that I spend unhappy about my body   _____

Average number of minutes I waste trying to find "skinny" clothes   _____

Average number of minutes I spend wondering what others
think about me   _____

Total minutes for one day   _____

Minutes above divided by 60   _____

**Hours above multiplied by 365
days**   _____

I can't tell you if the number of hours you spend every year focused on your weight is too high. Only you can determine how many moments of your life you want to give to your food. Only your friends and family can tell you what you are missing out on. Only God knows the wonderful things you can accomplish for Him when you leave this burden behind. You need to take a little time and *think* about your time.

When I weighed three hundred pounds, the seventy-three hundred hours I wasted on my obesity was a tragedy. I can't think of any other way to describe it. They represent lost opportunities, missed memories, and unfulfilled potential. I still mourn what I foolishly wasted, and this number hurts me more than the number on the scale ever did.

I believe your individual brain mass index is vital information in determining if you need this book. If your number is too high, you've probably been on countless diet and exercise plans in the past. Maybe none of them have been successful, or maybe you lost the weight for a period of time and put some, all, or even more of the weight back on. And what was the impact on your wallet?

In this book we are going to focus on the external pressures that can make reaching and staying at a healthy weight more difficult. There are messages to hear and messages to ignore. Want a quick preview? "The Lord doesn't love you less because you have love handles around your waist."

I want to ask you a few final questions before we move on. Are you ready to lose weight like a grown-up? Be a good steward of both your body and your finances? Have some wisdom about your food? If you want to claim the precious hours of your life back, you are holding the right book. Let's give your weight-loss journey a strong, running start.

The Whole Truth—So Help Me God

It can be easy to beat yourself up over the time you've lost agonizing over your weight. Even now I sometimes wonder what I missed during those seventy-three hundred hours I gave to my obesity. It can leave me in a pitiful pile of tears and self-loathing if I let it. Over the ast few years I've begun to look at my past mistakes like a bolt of electricity. Will it be crippling, or could it be illuminating instead? An uncontrolled bolt of electricity can burn me and leave me paralyzed. That same bolt of electricity can give me amazing energy to move forward if I harness it for good. There is no doubt that our past struggles and failures have power. Decide today what to do with that power.

House Call With Steve Hanor, MD

Question: You had quite a wake-up call about the foods you were eating and the affect those foods were having inside your body. How did that happen?

Dr. Hanor: In 2003 my mother died suddenly of a heart attack at age seventy. Her brother had died in his early fifties. At the time I was forty-nine and figured my heart attack would come at about the age of sixty…if I was lucky. Since I am a general internist (and a bad patient), I put myself on Lipitor to postpone my inevitable heart attack. I took medication off and on until 2007 when a friend of mine told me he was eating the *Eat to Live* way. I read the book but was not ready to plunge in until November of 2007 when my cholesterol came back at 278. An optimal LDL number is below 100 with an HDL number above 60 and triglycerides of less than 150.

The next day I fixed myself a large bowl of bean soup and added a lot of broccoli to the soup. My wife thought I was crazy, but soon realized I was serious. She was fairly willing to go on a high-nutrient eating style if it meant keeping me around longer. I have done well on this new eating style.

Question: Once you reached a healthier weight, did your diet go back to "normal"?

Dr. Hanor: No. My definition of normal has completely changed. We continue to eat a lot of vegetables (raw, steamed, and in soups), fruit, beans, nuts, and seeds. The diet is never boring, and we are always trying new things. My weight has gone from 205 to 172, and I have kept the weight off. My BMI is a little over 22, and my cholesterol has gone as low as 163.

With this diet a person tries to flood one's body with micro-nutrients. This can prevent and treat a wide range of illnesses. I have spent the last few years trying to share this information with as many patients as possible.

Steve Hanor, MD, is a general internist in Tennessee. With a history of heart disease in his family, Dr. Hanor radically changed his diet and his opinion about the way we should eat. He is a walking example for his patients of what can happen when we eat foods that are "less messed with" by human hands.

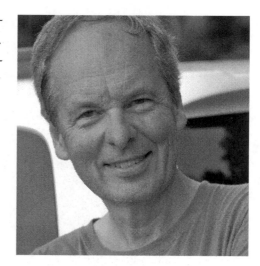

Chapter Three

COUNTING AND CLEANING

I F YOU ARE overweight, I'm going to tell you something that probably won't be much of a news flash. Losing weight is as simple (and as hard) as burning more calories than you eat. There are countless plans on the market that will take your money and give you advice on how to solve this daily math problem. Some have monthly fees in exchange for advice and recipes. Some plans will even precook your food and ship it right to your door—for a hefty price. The promise is that a smaller body is possible if you will just open your wallet.

The purpose of the Skinny Budget Diet is to give you something better than a quick fix to lose twenty pounds "before the big reunion." This is going to be an affordable, healthy relationship between you and your food. Wonder if it is possible? I remember being morbidly obese and believing that I couldn't lose weight. Let's shine a light on that myth right now.

BLAME IT ON METABOLISM

Eight years ago I was hoping to have a disease. No, not hoping to be *cured* of a disease. I wanted to be *diagnosed* with a disease. It is actually a common attitude among the morbidly obese.

Please don't misunderstand me. I didn't want to actually suffer. I didn't want cancer, heart disease, or diabetes. But when I weighed three hundred pounds, I wanted to be diagnosed with hypothyroidism. It was going to be my "magic bullet" for weight loss. I thought, "Just write me a prescription for levothyroxine and watch my pounds melt away."

Let's stop at this point for another quick and painless science lesson. Our thyroid is a gland located in the front of the neck just below the voice box (larynx). It releases hormones that control metabolism. Those with hypothyroidism don't produce enough thyroid hormone and can suffer from depression, fatigue, joint or muscle pain, constipation, thin/brittle hair, a puffy face, and unintentional weight gain. It's not "the look" that most of us would desire.

During my failed attempt to qualify for gastric bypass surgery, my primary care physician ordered a TSH (thyroid-stimulating hormone) blood test. There was no point in going through a risky weight-loss surgery if a faulty thyroid was to blame for my obesity. I'm sure that I calmly nodded my head when she explained the test. Below the neck I had every finger and toe crossed that my doctor would tell me that I had broken glands.

You can probably guess how this story ends. My thyroid was functioning just fine. Rats! I had fatigue because I was carrying 155 extra pounds on my body. I had a puffy face because I was carrying 155 extra pounds on my body. I had joint pain because I was carrying 155 extra pounds on my body. The thin and brittle hair? I'll blame that on genetics and the invention of the flat iron.

If you have several of the symptoms for hypothyroidism, it is important to see a physician and discuss the testing options. Reaching and maintaining a healthy weight for most of us is a matter of burning more calories than we eat. That is a tough order for those with hypothyroidism. When your body doesn't produce the proper amount of thyroid hormone, weight gain can be the result. In everyday language your "burn" doesn't have enough heat.

I read an article by James Norman, MD, FACE (Fellow of the American College of Endocrinology), to get a better picture of how widespread hypothyroidism is in this country. He reports that approximately ten million Americans have been diagnosed with a thyroid hormone deficiency, and as many as 10 percent of American woman have some degree of deficiency.[1] It sounds like a large number until we realize that a recent Gallup-Healthways Well-Being Index showed that 63.1 percent of adults in the US are categorized as either overweight or obese.[2] When we do the math, it is clear that there are a lot of healthy thyroids walking around inside of big bodies.

So if blaming our glands can't be used as an excuse for most of us, there is another concept on which to hang our extra pounds. Meet the set point theory.[3] This idea first started getting headlines in the 1980s. Scientists wondered if every human body has a natural weight—a size that our body quietly fights to reach and maintain. This concept was welcomed news for those lucky people who could eat whatever they want and not gain weight. The rest of us? Our outlook was mixed. We were told:

1. **If this planet ever suffers a global famine, our heavier set point will keep us alive.** Our skinny friends will be nothing but a memory. (I was always jealous of my friends who were thin, but not to the point of praying for famine.)

2. **Losing weight could be difficult for us because our bodies can't tell the difference between dieting and starvation.** Its ultimate goal is to store fat for that dreadful day when the supermarket shelves are empty. When we try to lower our calories and food intake, our bodies fight back by defending their fat stores. This is why so many dieters would struggle to keep the weight off... gaining and losing the same forty pounds.

3. **Experts also told us that we can "trick" our set point by increasing our exercise and level of activity.** We want our bodies to believe that we need

fuel to burn today. (Forget about a global famine; we need access to those fat reserves right now.)

The recent spike in obesity rates is making the set point idea a tough pill to swallow. Over the last twenty-five years our country has become dramatically heavier. Why the sudden rise in America's set point? Could it be that the body's desire to stay at a certain weight is no match for a high-calorie diet and sedentary lifestyle? And why do other countries see a rise in obesity rates when introduced to Western-style foods and larger portion sizes?

FATE VS. FREEDOM

Americans have a love affair with the concept of freedom. We fought to achieve it. We made it the cornerstone of our constitution. We continue to defend it. This fascination with being free doesn't end on the steps of the capitol. Think about the milestones we celebrate as a family and a community: baptism, graduation, wedding, and the birth of a child. Those big moments are simply an expression of our freedom to choose a path for our lives.

It is in this spirit of rugged individualism I ask my next questions: Do you blame bad genes or a slow metabolism when weight-loss plans don't work? Do you feel powerless? Do you believe fate gave you a body that can't be a healthy size?

For a country that enjoys so many freedoms, Americans are quick to give up our right to choose when it comes to our waistlines. We believe that our obesity is beyond our control. Instead of taking a hard look at our food choices, we want doctors to give us an excuse for our extra weight. Just order me an "It's Not My Fault" T-shirt, size 4X please. When I weighed three hundred pounds, I actually *wanted* a disease to explain away my obesity. It would have been a relief to hear that fate had dealt me a bad genetic hand.

As much as it hurts, it's important to start any weight-loss plan with the truth. I don't know your specific medical situation, but here are the facts for a *vast* majority of us:

1. **It is possible that you are genetically programmed to carry a few extra pounds or that you simply have a large frame.** This is why physicians have a weight range for "normal" that is fairly wide. Beware of anyone who tells you that you must be at one specific number for your height. As a woman who is five feet, eight inches tall, my healthy weight can fall between 122 and 169 pounds. There is a lot of room for individuality in that range.

2. **The bigger you are, the more calories you will burn.** If a 150-pound person and a 250-pound person walk on a treadmill at the same speed and incline for twenty minutes, the 250-pound person will burn more calories. Larger people even burn more calories at rest!

3. **We have extra pounds because we are eating more calories than our bodies need to carry out their daily functions.** The good news? We have the power to change this and get to a healthier size. The bad news? We must take responsibility and stop blaming our glands.

As you begin the Skinny Budget Diet, I want you to celebrate the freedom God gave you to own your weight. Fate isn't as powerful as we would like to believe. For most of us our size is the direct result of the choices we make every day. I'm going to guide you into some good ones.

THE GUTS TO LOSE THE GUT

"He had a broad face and a little round belly that shook when he laughed like a bowlful of jelly." Get ready, Santa. We are going to examine that round belly, and we may decide to update *'Twas the Night Before Christmas* for the twenty-first century. We could make it more accurate if it read something like this: "He had a broad face and a little round belly that shook when he laughed like metabolically active visceral fat." Just rolls off the tongue, doesn't it?

The good news is that there is time to lose some jelly in the belly before Santa springs to his sleigh once more. Studies show that the stomach is actually first in line for fat burning. Endocrinologists and obesity researchers at the Mayo Clinic found that the majority of dieters lost weight in the abdominal region before anywhere else.[4] Your belly will start shrinking even before your face gets thinner or your ankles come out from hiding.

If you need additional proof that we are wonderfully made, this might be it. God gave us an intelligent fat-burning oven. Instead of initially going after the subcutaneous fat right below the skin, our bodies almost always target the visceral fat first. This stuff lies deep inside the abdomen and surrounds many of our organs. It is biochemically different from subcutaneous fat and is metabolized by the liver.

Physicians have found that excessive amounts of visceral fat can produce hormones and other substances that raise blood pressure, change our good and bad cholesterol levels, and impair our ability to use insulin. In my active imagination I picture this dangerous fat crowding out our other organs, feeding them poison, and interfering with their important work within our bodies. An overabundance of visceral fat is that life threatening.

So now that we have identified the enemy, how are we going to remove it? It is one of the questions I am asked most often when I speak with groups about weight loss. There is a vast amount of misinformation and more than a few greedy companies that use our desperation to make a quick buck. Let's look for the truth and see if we have the guts to lose the gut.

1. Belly-burning foods—fact or fiction?

The answer to this question is yes. It is both fact and fiction. After extensive reading and interviewing several registered dieticians, I can report that there is no food that will magically melt belly fat. If we eat four thousand calories a day and never sweat in our sweatpants, eating five grapefruits before bed won't give us a smaller stomach. It will simply make us a sour bed partner.

But before you write off the power of food, there is some interesting research about whole grains. The *American Journal of Clinical Nutrition* published a study with two groups of obese individuals.[5] The first group was given a daily diet with whole grains plus five servings of fruits and vegetables, three servings of low-fat dairy, and two servings of lean meat. The second group was given the same diet but ate refined grains rather than whole grains. The first group lost more weight. Along with watching calories and portion sizes, researchers believe that whole grains can change our glucose and insulin response, making it easier for us to utilize fat stores.

The Tummy Take Home: Whole grains are one weapon in your fat-burning arsenal, but they can't single-handedly win your battle of the bulge. A bowl of whole-grain cereal is a healthy start to your morning. Don't expect it to cancel out the rest of your day if your diet also includes large portions of pasta, pistachio ice cream, and Pringles. Calories still count.

2. Belly fat–melting exercises—fact or fiction?

Again, the answer is yes. Sit-ups, crunches, and abdominal machines may help you build muscle, but they can't specifically target and burn the layer of fat around those muscles.

When I see people at my gym torturing themselves with endless crunches, it's hard to keep my mouth shut. If these individuals are eating too many calories, they may never see the beautiful abdominal muscles they are struggling to sculpt. Does this mean that exercise is a waste of time in your mission to have a smaller waist? No, we just need to focus about six inches higher with the heart.

Cardiovascular exercises that increase your heart rate will burn fat everywhere in your body, including the abdominal area. These can be activities such as walking, riding a bike, swimming, running, dancing, and using elliptical or stair-climbing machines.

Exercises that use weights and resistance can also help burn fat. Muscle mass diminishes with age. Strength training can reverse this process, giving us more muscle and a bigger "calorie-burning oven" at any age. Our body meets this extra demand for energy by utilizing fat stores. And if we have too much "potential energy" around the stomach area, that fat is generally first in line for the oven.

The Tummy Take Home: If it has been a long time since you've put on a pair of tennis shoes, get a green light from your doctor before you begin an exercise plan. I had to start slow. My goal when I weighed three hundred pounds was to walk for forty-five minutes at least four days a week. It helped me lose weight faster and feel stronger. (More on this coming up in chapter 4.)

3. Belly-shrinking drugs—fact or fiction?

This one is fiction. Unless the FDA surprises us next week with approval on SRT1720 or some other metabolism-boosting drug, there is no such thing as a pill that will lower your number on the scale without some effort or sweat equity on your part.

The Tummy Take Home: With 60 percent of American adults either considered overweight or obese, I understand our desire to find a cure for the Santa belly. I understand that losing extra fat will greatly reduce our risk for diseases such as heart attacks, strokes, diabetes, cancer, and even dementia. And within my own body I finally understand how it feels to climb a flight of stairs without knee pain.

When I look at all the health benefits that could come from a miracle diet pill, I still hope that one is never invented. I don't want to see an entire generation that is thin on the outside and sick on the inside. I don't want a world where bingeing on empty calories has no cost. There may be less weight gain, but there will also be a lot less nutrition. Why bother to fill your plate with color? Why think about vitamins, minerals, and lean protein? Just pop a pill and eat all the tan and white carbohydrates you want.

It doesn't give us a warm and fuzzy feeling to think about, but God created our bodies to get fat when we make poor eating choices. He wants us to see and feel the consequences of our decisions. He wants to get our attention. It felt like a divine punishment the day that my scale hit three hundred pounds. Looking back, that consequence was really a love letter.

The Lord was not so gently showing me that my definition of eating was actually an addiction. He wants our food to sustain us and give us life—not be a slow form of suicide. If you are struggling to button your jeans, God may be trying to tell you something.

Where Cravings End and Hunger Pains Begins

Pain isn't fun. We will go to great lengths to avoid it. And even with all that effort, most of us are fascinated by the concept of pain. Twisted but true. Women love to share their tales of drama and daring from the delivery room. My youngest son, who weighed twelve pounds and four ounces at birth, will earn me serious pain points from the other ladies in the room until I confess that he was born through cesarean section. Without the built-in suffering of childbirth men can still join the pain party by passing kidney stones the size of golf balls, falling off the roof while hanging Christmas lights, and other acts of courage.

My favorite is a true story straight from my own house. My husband and his friends spent five minutes of their lives (*time that they will never get back*) discussing how much money it would take before they would be willing to wrestle a raccoon barehanded. I believe that the potential loss of one or two fingers drove the final dollar amount into the thousands.

Avoiding a cage match with wild animals is generally wise; avoiding pain at all costs is not. Pain is the body's way of getting the brain's attention. It is an early warning system. We don't often thank God for the gift of pain, but we would have a much shorter life expectancy if the Lord didn't give us the ability to feel it.

During the twenty years of my obesity, I had two pregnancies, one defective gallbladder, and a lot of joint pain due to my three-hundred-pound body. And even with all that discomfort going around, there was one pain I can't ever remember experiencing when I was heavy—hunger pain. I ate so often and in such large amounts that my stomach never had the opportunity to legitimately grumble for food. Intense cravings and an overactive appetite gave me a busy belly that never felt empty.

This practice of pre-feeding is common among the obese. Many of the overweight men and women I speak to have lived for years without feeling an empty stomach. We might forget to have the oil changed in our cars or stay up to date on our tetanus shots, but we never forget to feed the cravings. It is high on our daily priority list.

Before we define the difference between a hunger pain and a food craving, I'd like to go back to the anatomy classroom for some tummy tutorials. Some of these facts surprised me.

The Stomach 101

1. The average adult stomach is about twelve inches long and six inches wide. The stomach's capacity is about one quart.

2. The size of the stomach does not correlate with weight or weight control. People who are naturally thin can have the same size or even larger stomachs than people who battle their weight throughout

a lifetime. "Weight has nothing to do with the size of the stomach. In fact, even people who have had stomach-reducing surgeries, making their tummy no larger than a walnut, can override the small size and still gain weight," says Dr. Joseph Levy, a gastroenterologist at NYU.[6]

3. Once you are an adult, your stomach pretty much remains the same size (*unless you have surgery to intentionally make it smaller*). "Eating less won't shrink your stomach," says Dr. Mark Moyad, director of preventive and alternative medicine at the University of Michigan's Medical Center in Ann Arbor. Moyad does say that eating less can help us reset our "appetite thermostat" and make it easier to stick with a weight-loss plan.[7]

When I started my final weight-loss plan in 2007, my mouth had to give my stomach a little tough love. It was necessary for me to experience the tugging cramps of what an empty stomach actually felt like. When I lowered my calories from 5,000 a day to 2,000 a day, I had hunger pains from time to time. They were the strongest about an hour before lunch and dinner and felt more like pangs than actual pain.

After years of dreading an empty stomach, I am pleased to report that a little hunger didn't kill me, make me wish that I were dead, or inspire me to kill anyone else. It simply made my meals taste better and helped me make the important distinction between a craving and a true need to give my body fuel. That difference made all the difference during my 155-pound weight loss. Not all of the messages coming out of our brains deserve a response in our mouths.

Cravings 101

If you think that an overactive appetite for junk food is in your head, you are right. Numerous studies show that the areas of the brain responsible for memory and sensing pleasure can contribute to our food cravings. Here is what the research is showing:

1. Three regions of the brain (*the hippocampus, insula, and caudate*) are activated during food-craving episodes. Brain tests at the Monell Chemical Senses Center suggest that "memory areas of the brain (which are responsible for associating a specific food with a reward) are actually more important to food cravings than the brain's reward center."[8]

2. "Blocking the opiate receptors in the brain, which sense pleasure, can blunt a person's desire to eat foods rich in fat and sugar," according to research by Adam Drewnowski, PhD, of the University of Washington.[9]

3. Carbohydrates can boost our levels of the hormone serotonin and give us a feeling of calm. So why don't we crave the carbohydrates found in fruits and whole grains rather than the carbohydrates found in cherry pies and potato chips? Researchers did some investigating by "stressing out" a group of rats.

Scientists from University of California at San Francisco put rats in a high-stress environment and discovered that fearful rats preferred to eat foods high in sugar and fat.[10] When the rats ate these "souped-up carbs," their brains produced less of the stress-related hormones that trigger the fight-or-flight response.[11] The rats self-medicated their anxiety with sugar and fat.

I admit I have some mixed feelings about sharing this research with you. We can walk away from all the science with an attitude that our cravings and daily food choices are beyond our control. If that were true, I would still weigh three hundred pounds or maybe be approaching three hundred fifty at this point.

God didn't create us to be puppets under the complete control of the chemical strings in our brains. The food cravings that feel so strong at the beginning of a diet diminish significantly as the pounds come off. During the first two months of my weight loss, I had to take out a restraining order on doughnuts and keep them at least five hundred yards from my kitchen. My desire to eat half the box was too strong. Doughnuts can now sit on my counter for an entire weekend, and I don't have the desire to eat even one. Every time you feel a craving but don't feed the craving, you will get stronger.

The walk toward this type of true authority over your food requires an accurate map. You must know where you are right now in order to travel in the right direction and reach your destination. I want you to honestly answer these questions: How many calories did you eat yesterday? Can you even give an educated guess that would be within five hundred calories of what you actually consumed? And how many calories should someone your weight, height, age, and gender eat to lose one to two pounds a week?

Don't feel discouraged if you don't know the answer to that question. Remember that my guess was more than two thousand calories off when I actually wrote down my "Day in the Life" menu. It can be tricky to remember every roll, every teaspoon of mayo, and every cookie, but it is a critical piece of information.

LET'S START TRACKING

Before waking up and announcing, "Today, I will start my weight loss," we're going to begin by knowing your calorie target. It's easy. Eat what you would normally eat and track your calories for one week. Don't alter your portion sizes, but pay attention. Get a good idea of how many teaspoons, cups, and pounds of food you are eating.

For all of you diet "veterans" out there, I can almost see you rolling your eyes at this point and muttering, "Tracking calories? Forget about it. I've tried this before, and I don't have time to write down every bite." Just hang on. Calorie watching has moved into the twenty-first century, and it is a lot easier than it used to be.

There are free tools available online that can make recording your calories faster than the old "diet diary" with a pen and a piece of paper. You want to select a site with a database that can calculate the calories in common meals made at home, packaged foods from the grocery stores, and even restaurant dishes. It's important that the website you choose can track everything from meat loaf and mashed potatoes to Oreo cookies and a Big Mac. There are a lot of options out there with the tools you will need, including some that have apps for your smartphone. Here are a few of the many free sites that I've found: www.sparkpeople.com or www.livestrong.com/thedailyplate.

If you are on your computer checking e-mail and Facebook, make a stop on your tracker as a part of your evening routine or enter it as you go through the day with the Internet application on your cell phone. Once you get the hang of it, recording your food should take less than ten minutes a day.

Don't think you can spare the time? Look at it this way: you are putting the minutes that you would normally spend wishing you were thinner to better use! Don't want to spend the rest of your life tracking calories? You won't. But in order to learn balance, we're going to put training wheels on this weight-loss plan. That is what counting calories will be for you during the first several weeks of this diet plan.

When you learn what a portion size really looks like, when your cravings for high-fat/high-sugar foods have diminished, and when you feel more at peace with your plate, the training wheels will come off and precise calorie counting will no longer be necessary.

You will have balance with your food. I haven't recorded my daily calories in three years, but it was essential during the early days of my weight loss.

A good calorie-tracking website should start by asking you to enter some vital statistics such as height, weight, age, and your average level of daily activity. Not only should it calculate how many calories you are currently eating and drinking, but it should also give you a target number in order to lose one to two pounds every week.

When calculating your daily calories, the food you are eating is only half of the equation. Look for a tracking website that will also allow you to enter your physical activities for the day. I could "earn back" calories for everything from vacuuming my house and walking around the neighborhood to weights and cardio machines. Don't forget to include your calories burned in your daily calorie mix.

Remember, we are only gathering information at this point. Unless you have the stomach flu, the calorie tracking website will probably tell you that you've eaten too many calories to hit your daily target. That is OK. We are taking a journey, and you can't travel to where you want to go if you don't know where you are right now.

Why is all this information so important?

The fact that most diets fail in the first two weeks may not be surprising to you, but the reason for the diet failures may be. I always thought that my diets didn't work because I was still eating too much food. Looking back, I believe I struggled for twenty years because I was trying to fall from five thousand calories a day to something around fifteen hundred. I thought that was the magic number to lose weight, and it was a crucial mistake.

The daily calorie goal of someone who weighs one hundred forty pounds is much different than what my target should have been at three hundred pounds. I was trying to cut 70 percent of my daily calories overnight. Of course, I was frustrated and thought I was starving. I'm sure I was also as mean as a snake. I quit many of my past diet plans because I was setting completely unrealistic calorie goals.

As a woman who was five feet, eight inches tall and weighed 300 pounds, I could actually eat 2,385 calories a day and lose 1.5 pounds each week. When I started my weight-loss plan in 2007, I learned that 2,385 calories is *a lot* of food if you make smart choices.

When the weight started to fall, my target number of daily calories went down, but it went down slowly. It wasn't a 75 percent drop in calories that made me want to commit petty larceny on my kid's Christmas candy. Take the time to calculate your own individual number. Again, we want to go on this journey with a good map of where we are and where we want to be.

HOW OFTEN SHOULD YOU RING THE DINNER BELL?

If you were born before Ronald and Nancy Reagan moved into the White House, chances are that you grew up with parents who believed in spanking, no swimming immediately after eating, and no snacking between meals. Dentists were never any help. They were firmly on the side of our parents in this "between meals" debate.

My family dentist actually gave out pencils at Halloween instead of candy. Every year my sister and I were encouraged to climb this dentist's driveway just to be rewarded with a plain, yellow #2 pencil. That always seemed wrong to me.

Fast-forward a few decades. Spanking is controversial in some circles, and physicians now claim that we can swim after eating with no increased risk of drowning. So what about snacking? Is a "three meals a day" schedule obsolete in the twenty-first century?

The answer to that question depends completely on you. I want to present both sides of this argument and ask you to honestly examine your eating patterns. This isn't the time to dream about the way you wish you could eat. The purpose of this is to discover the ideal way for you to receive a steady stream of energy. Eating between meals can save a weight-loss plan for some and kill it for others.

Group one: The Three Squares

When we sit down for a meal, we have a picture in our minds of how it should look. For the Three Squares, an ideal plate might have meat, potatoes and/or bread, vegetables, and dessert. Throw in a cup of coffee or sweet tea, and this group is in business. If you are a Three Squares, you grew up with the belief that a good child always cleans his/her plate. That belief is still with you.

Not sure if you are a Three Squares? Think back to your eating last week, and let's see what we discover:

1. Did you generally eat everything on your plate and go back for more?

2. Do you crave food that is warm?

3. Do you enjoy lingering around the table after a meal?

4. When you snack between meals, is it because you crave something sweet, salty, crunchy, etc.?

5. Are your go-to snacks generally higher fat carbohydrates? (This is a group rich in "C," and I don't mean vitamin C. Think candy, cake, cookies, and chips.)

If you answered yes to at least three of the questions above, you are most likely a Three Squares. Weight loss for you is achievable, but snacks between meals should be very light in calories. Because of that ideal "meal picture" in your head, you will be most comfortable if 70–80 percent of your daily recommended calories come from three meals a day. This will allow you to have meat, potatoes/bread, vegetables, and dessert without feeling deprived. Your family can continue to have meals where everyone lingers around the table.

Weight loss for you is all about making smart decisions when your elbows hit the table. You will need to:

1. **Know how many calories you can eat every day to lose one to two pounds a week.** This number is unique to you. If you are a big guy, you might be able to eat 800 calories at each meal and slowly lose weight. For most of us that number is lower.

2. **Look for smart switches in the kitchen.** You can still have your potatoes and bread, but read the nutritional information. Maybe a baked potato has fewer calories than mashed. Maybe a roll has fewer calories than a cheesy bread stick. Know how many calories are in each item.

3. **Watch those portion sizes.** There is no shame in pulling out a measuring cup when you first start your weight-loss plan. Your eyes and your brain are learning something new.

4. **Plate your food in the kitchen (with a measuring cup in hand) and walk away.** Don't torture yourself by putting a heaping plate of biscuits on your dining room table!

5. **Don't overcook.** I'm not talking about temperature here. It's important to prepare only the amount of food needed for the crowd you are feeding. If you need only four hamburgers, don't grill six. This is the mistake that I made for years. Not only was I wasting money, but also I was giving myself an excuse to overeat. I didn't want the food, but it seemed like a sin to throw it away.

Group two: The Happy Snacker

I am a member of this group. At three hundred pounds, my daily calories were a combination of breakfast, lunch, dinner (because I grew up believing that three meals a day is next to godliness), and several snacks that were also large in size. Not surprisingly the result was obesity and a woman who was really confused about how to eat.

I don't think I'm alone here. Wondering if you are a Happy Snacker, too? Think back to your meals last week, and let's see what we can find:

1. Did you eat fairly "normal" portion sizes at dinner...only to eat an hour later?

2. Are you happy with both warm and cold foods?

3. When you are finished eating a meal, are you ready to get out of your chair and move on?

4. When you snack between meals, is it sometimes because you feel drained of energy or just plain crabby?

5. Are your go-to snacks a little more complicated? (Think peanut butter sandwiches, bowls of cereal, and slices of pizza.)

If you answered yes to at least three of the questions above, you might be a Happy Snacker. Welcome to the club! Weight loss for us starts with the knowledge that three square meals a day don't work for us. We can still sit down with our families for dinner, but our plates will look a little different. Get ready for comments such as, "Is that all you are eating for dinner?" The people who love us need to understand that our calories are spread out during the day. We aren't starving!

Weight loss for us involves making smart decisions (*and a lot of them*) during the hours that we are awake:

1. **Know how many calories you should eat to lose one to two pounds a week.** This is true for us too. If you aren't sure, visit a free site such as www .livestrong.com/thedailyplate or www.sparkpeople .com and quickly get your individual number.

2. **Do a nutrition check.** Our meals are smaller, but we still need to finish the day with the right amount of fuel. Our 10:00 a.m. bowl of cereal might be a good source of vitamins, calcium, and fiber. Our 2:30 p.m. turkey and veggie sandwich can be an ideal source for protein and even more vitamins.

3. **Watch those portion sizes.** This is a must for the Happy Snackers. If oversized portions can hurt a weight-loss plan for the Three Squares, it can kill our plan because we are eating more often during the day. If you are someone who has trouble eating a small amount and stopping, frequent meals isn't your plan. Stick with the Three Squares.

4. **Plate your food in the kitchen and walk away.** We don't want temptations on our tables either.

5. **Use your body as a guide.** If it's time for your mid-morning "mini meal" and you aren't hungry, that's OK. Pay attention, and don't go more than an hour past your hunger pangs.

So are you a Three Squares or a Happy Snacker? Both groups have their challenges, and both groups can shed the pounds. Getting to a healthy weight (and staying there) starts with "knowing thy stomach" and also "knowing thy brain." This is just one of many reasons why the prepackaged, one-plan-fits-all approach to weight loss doesn't work. You are unique. Your weight-loss plan will be too.

I Eat. Therefore, I Snack.

What are your favorite treats? That may sound like a strange thing to ask when you are starting a weight-loss plan. In a perfect world we would eat perfectly nutritional food providing us with the perfect balance of vitamins, minerals, and protein. Foods containing empty calories and saturated fat would taste perfectly awful. I don't know about you, but perfection has always been slightly out of my reach. "I eat. Therefore, I snack."

Before day one of your Skinny Budget Diet use your online tracker to write a "go to" snack list in your journal. This step can actually be a lot of fun. Write down each item, the serving size, the number of calories in each serving, and if it can travel. A container of yogurt can be a great snack, but it won't work during an eight-hour car trip without a way to keep it cold.

If you live with a spouse or children, you are going to make a second snack list with the help of your family. Write down the little treats they enjoy. This could be doughnuts with chocolate frosting on Sunday morning, Oreo cookies in a lunch box, a bowl of cookie dough ice cream after dinner, and so on. Spend some time with this, and make the list as long as possible. Don't forget to include drinks on this list—soda, iced coffees, energy drinks, wine, etc. They can all contain calories and need to be examined.

After both lists are complete, cross off the items that are irresistible to you. Need a definition of irresistible? If you consume several servings in a one- or two-day period and would still eat more, it is irresistible. These food and drink items will not come into your house during your weight loss. (You might need to cross items off of the list away from the eyes of your children!)

When I weighed three hundred–plus pounds, I liked cinnamon

rolls, and I *loved* chocolate doughnuts. The cinnamon rolls stayed on my son's Sunday morning breakfast list because I can walk away from a cinnamon roll. It was a once-a-week treat that gave him a break from the cereal and fruit he generally ate for the other six days out of the week. The doughnuts, on the other hand, were banished from my house for the first year of my weight loss. Sorry, son!

What will make the cut and be a "go to" snack for you? Here are some questions to ask yourself before you put an item down on your list:

1. **Can I eat one serving a day and stop, or will it keep "whispering" for me to eat more?** This is the million-dollar question when it comes to snacking. In the beginning of your weight-loss plan you may underestimate the "power" of certain snacks. Before every trip to the grocery store look back at your eating. Did that friendly miniature candy bar with only 80 calories become a not-so-miniature calorie bomb when you ate five in one day? It might need to be replaced with another snack idea.

2. **Is there a lower-calorie version of this snack available?** There are 250 calories in a 1.74 ounce bag of peanut M&Ms. A slightly smaller 1.14 ounce bag of pretzel M&Ms only has 150 calories. In moderation both can be a satisfying snack in my opinion. If you replace your daily bag of peanut M&Ms with a bag of pretzel M&Ms, you will eat 36,500 fewer calories after one year. That could equal ten less pounds on your scale! Many online calorie tracking websites will actually recommend "lighter" versions of the snacks you are researching.

3. **Does this snack also provide me with some good nutrition?** When you are writing down the calories of your favorite snacks, you might be tempted to leave off items such as nuts. For most varieties two ounces will add up to more than 300 calories. But before you completely banish snacks such as nuts from your house, understand that the nutrition and "feeling full" power of these snacks may make them worth the calorie investment for you.

Nuts are rich in unsaturated fats and are some of the richest sources of protein in the plant kingdom. Nuts also contain fiber and phytosterols. These nutrients have been shown to lower cholesterol. Do a little bit of research and watch your portion sizes. For example, half a cup of macadamia nuts will run about 467 calories, while half a cup of pistachios is about 317 calories. There is no reason that snacks such as nuts can't be on your "go to" list as also being healthy for your weight-loss plan.

I ate snacks from day one of my weight loss. I tell you this because too many of us picture "the diet" as being the place where fun foods go to die. Believe me, losing weight is challenging enough without believing that you will never enjoy food or eat sugar again. Don't despair. Your snacks will live on!

Your Initiation Into the Breakfast Club

If you want to start a fight at your next dinner party, bring up the subject of breakfast. I thought topics such as religion and politics were touchy, but it is nothing compared to the heated discussions you will hear about the first meal of the day. Passions run high on both sides of the alarm clock.

Breakfast is grrrrreat! This is the "must break your fast" crowd. I won't keep you in suspense. I am a card-carrying member of the breakfast club. My family of four currently has in its kitchen:

bacon, ham, eggs from a local farm, pancake/waffle mix, fresh fruit, cinnamon rolls, raisin bread, bagels, oatmeal, bran, two varieties of toaster pastries, three varieties of granola/fiber/protein bars, and four different types of breakfast cereals (from the very bland to the amazingly colorful). Whew! We who love breakfast really love breakfast.

Breakfast is grrrrrross! This is the "you can't make me" eat breakfast crowd. I had no idea that these people even existed until I went to college. It turns out that they are everywhere. The first meal of the day for this group is a cup of coffee followed by some toothpaste. If you are in the anti-breakfast club, skipping this meal might be the result of a busy morning schedule or a desire to lose weight. Others just need a few hours of sunlight to give their appetites a chance to wake up.

Most physicians recommend that we eat some healthy protein, vitamins, and fiber before we walk out the door in the morning. And before you ask, supplements (even ones as tasty as Flintstones chewables) can't take the place of real food. So when I first started speaking with groups about nutrition and weight loss, I was surprised at all the breakfast questions that came up: "Do I have to eat breakfast?" "Can I wait an hour or two before I eat it?" "Will skipping breakfast make me gain weight?"

And to these questions I have this insightful answer. It depends. Let's start with the idea that breakfast must be at the top of our morning to-do list. Should we turn off our alarm clocks and immediately reach for Tony the Tiger and Jimmy Dean? I've heard the arguments in favor of this. Unless you are a midnight snacker, most of us have gone eight to ten hours without food. That's technically a fast. I agree that it is important to give our bodies some quality fuel after such a long period, but I think there is room here for common sense.

Not everyone has big appetite first thing in the morning. That's OK. If the idea of an early breakfast makes your stomach turn, wait an hour or two before eating. Don't choke something down just for the sake of refueling. Food shouldn't be torture, and you are more likely to eat breakfast consistently if it is enjoyable. Another trick for the morning squeamish is to start slow. It will still qualify as breakfast even if you can't eat 500 calories in one sitting. Go with something light, and move into the higher protein foods after you've rubbed the sleep out of your eyes.

At this point I can almost hear a few of you out there saying, "Fine advice for some people, but I don't have time for breakfast. My morning schedule is too crazy." I've been there. Who am I kidding? I'm still there. The hectic rush to pack school lunches, supervise last-minute homework, and find missing tennis shoes is real. If you are committed to giving this breakfast thing a try, I have some tips that might help.

1. **Plan the night before.** This doesn't just apply to your breakfast menu. Our goal is to find ten or fifteen precious minutes in your morning. Look at your entire morning routine. Have your clothes, shoes, backpacks, homework, permission slips, cell phones, car keys, and so on ready to walk out the door. Not only will you find the time to eat in the morning, but it also might actually be the most relaxing meal of the day.

2. **Think about what you really like to eat and be willing to experiment.** There are countless microwave and toaster breakfast options in the grocery stores. Most take less than two minutes to prepare. Honestly, I'm not a big fan of how they taste, but the men in my family are. You might be too. Remember to read those labels, and look for lean protein and fiber without too much salt. You'll want to avoid eating 50 percent of your daily allowance of sodium before the rooster crows.

3. **Don't put yourself in a "cereal" box.** As far as I
   know, there is no such thing as the breakfast police.
   Last night's leftovers can make a great breakfast.
   Ever tried a slice of last night's veggie pizza? Good
   stuff! If you can handle the tomato sauce, peppers,
   and onions early in the morning, it makes a tasty
   a.m. meal. Some people skip breakfast because they
   don't like traditional breakfast foods. No problem.
   Just call it brunch and heat up last night's dinner.
   We won't tell.

And now ladies and gentlemen, it's time. I've danced around the
million-dollar question long enough. Let's answer this once and for
all. Will avoiding breakfast lead to weight gain? On the surface the
idea sounds illogical. We are cutting calories out of our day. How
can that be bad? Isn't less food the whole purpose of weight loss?
It is at this point that you need to examine the choices you are
making during the rest of your day. Ask yourself:

1. **When I skip breakfast, how do I feel around
   10:00 a.m.?** Am I dreaming of the oversized portions I'll get at lunch? Do I give up and hit the
   vending machine to keep me going? And as a side
   note, doctors have found that long periods without
   food (twelve hours or more) can increase a body's
   insulin response. Experts say that this response also
   increases our fat storage and leads to weight gain.

2. **Am I eating quality food?** If I skip breakfast, how
   colorful is the rest of my day? Is my food always
   white, tan, or brown? It's interesting, but people who
   eat breakfast tend to make better food choices for
   lunch and dinner. Those pesky experts have found
   that when we skip breakfast, we are more likely to
   skip our colorful fruits and vegetables too.

3. How is my energy level? Am I half asleep every afternoon? Do I skip exercise when I skip meals? Physical activity requires fuel—strong, reliable, consistent power.

We would never depend on a flashlight that burns bright one minute and is dim the next. Too often we have lower expectations for our bodies than we do the ten-dollar gadgets in our garage. And too often we treat our machines with more care. Getting through the day requires fuel and making the effort to exercise requires even *more* fuel.

If you feel tired all the time, understand that it's not a part of the aging process. Your body is sending you a message. Pay attention to it.

LADIES, CAN WE TALK?

This might be the moment when I officially lose my girlie-girl card. I like buying presents. I like party games. And obviously I've liked more than a few pieces of cake in my life. But when you combine gifts, games (that too often involve toilet paper), and gooey frosting, the final result can be an event that strikes fear in the hearts of men. Get out your glitter and lace invitations, ladies. It's time for a shower.

I'm at a stage age in life where there seems to be a wedding or baby shower every weekend. Honestly I try to enjoy them. Newlyweds and new parents need our support. They need sage advice. They also desperately need supplies. I understand the purpose for throwing showers, and I'm grateful that there are women in the world who bravely organize these events. I just wish that my rump didn't always fall asleep after sitting in the same folding chair for two hours.

My husband believes I don't like wedding and baby showers because there are no men in the room. He might be right. The best shower I ever attended included the expectant father (who had the misfortune of opening a new breast pump in front of forty females). Good stuff!

In the spirit of gift giving, I would like to dedicate the following information to women everywhere who blow up balloons, cut radishes into little flowers, and painstakingly save every bow. It's time for a weight-loss shower. Guys, you are welcome to stay in the room, or you can watch *Shark Week* on the Discovery Channel and I'll see you in the next chapter.

Are the men gone? Let's grab a roll of toilet paper and start this party.

If you've attended a wedding or baby shower recently, perhaps you've noticed the miniature portion sizes. They always irritated me when I weighed three hundred pounds. Whose idea was it to take a decent size piece of cake, cut it into a billon little squares, and call it a petit four?

Most of us could eat a heaping plate of them, but we know that other women are watching. I don't think we ever outgrow peer pressure. So instead of eating ten petit fours, we eat two and talk about how full we are. I would wrap a handful of petit fours in a napkin to "take home to my husband." This will be news to him because the petit fours in my purse never made it all the way into the house.

Men eat much differently. Could you image a group of guys cutting bacon into tiny pieces, putting them on doilies, and calling them petit pigs? It would never happen. I believe there are biological reasons for this even beyond their instinctive aversion to doilies. Size does matter when we look at portion sizes.

According to the Centers for Disease Control and Prevention the average man in the United States is just under five feet ten inches tall and weighs 194.7 pounds. The average woman is just under five feet four inches tall and weighs 164.7 pounds.[12] Six inches and 30 pounds may not seem like a big difference when comparing the sexes, but the number of daily calories required for the average Joe and the average Jane are very different.

Let's start with Joe. If he is thirty years old and somewhat active, he should eat between 2,500 and 2,600 calories every day to stay at his current size. If Jane is thirty years old and classified as somewhat active, her daily calorie requirements to stay at her current size are between 1,900 and 2,000. The 600 extra calories given to the males can get females into some tummy trouble.

Married women are twice as likely to become obese when compared to single ladies who are the same age. I don't believe it is because we've caught a man and want to celebrate by "letting ourselves go." Married women spend billions of dollars annually on clothes, makeup, and accessories. Clearly we care how we look in the eyes of our husbands. It is how we look at our plates that can be the problem.

Think back to the last meal that you shared at home with your husband. Did each person fill his or her own plate? Did one person do the honors for both? Did you eat foods he loves and you think are just OK? These may seem like tiny details, but they can have a huge impact on your waistline. Here is what happened in my newlywed kitchen:

1. **When I grabbed the spatula, I automatically put the same amount of food on both plates**—even though my husband is four inches taller than me, has more muscle, and burns more calories in any given day than I do. My reason for dishing out man-sized portions probably sounded something like this: I worked hard today. I can eat as much as he can. Three cheers for equality!

2. **When my husband served our meals, he also put the same amount of food on both plates.** Guys don't want to hand us a dinner that looks too

skimpy. Who can blame them? Sensitive women everywhere would translate it as "my husband thinks I'm fat" or "my husband is trying to save money by starving me." Laugh if you want, but you know it's true.

3. **I began eating foods that were never a part of my diet when I was single.** My husband introduced me to several dishes, including fried potatoes, sweet and sour chicken, pork rinds, and crab rangoon. I enjoyed some of these new items. The pork rinds? I ate them simply because they were in the house. When I combined this mindless eating with the "equality" of my portion sizes, it isn't surprising that I gained one hundred pounds during the first five years of my marriage.

We are given a lot of advice at a wedding shower on how to build a relationship that lasts. Wise women tell us how to respect our husbands, how to pray for our husbands, and even the right way to fight with our husbands. No one tells us how to eat with our husbands. They should. Unless you are the same height and have the same muscle mass as your guy, equality has no place at your kitchen table.

Before puberty there isn't a significant difference in the muscle mass between males and females. All this changes once puberty kicks in. Men develop higher levels of testosterone. The result is a broader frame and increased muscle mass. Women see higher levels of estrogen. This gives us more body fat, less muscle and bone mass, and a lighter total weight than men.

And because these pages are all about the ladies, I can't end our weight-loss shower without a quick conversation about shoes. My husband wears a size 13. When I put one of his shoes against my size 8 pumps, there is no comparison. The man has much larger feet than I do.

Can you imagine how ridiculous it would be for me to wear his size 13 boots in the name of equality? Just thinking about it puts a blister on the back of my heel. Stomping around in his shoes would be silly and painful. Our needs are different. Our tastes are different, and our bodies are different. It's a fact I praise God for daily.

You might not always feel like a petite flower, but our portion sizes need to be more petite when compared to the guys. We aren't men, and we need to stop eating like we are. Save that second hamburger or that third slice of pizza for your hubby. He'll love you for it!

The Whole Truth—So Help Me God

I hesitated to put the word *diet* in the title of this book. It conjures up too many memories of rules and restrictions. Few people can have a healthy relationship with food based on stern laws and harsh punishments for infractions. Who wants to live that way? For the remainder of the book, understand that diet is simply defined as the foods and drinks we consume. We will count calories just long enough to learn what a portion size looks like and feels like in our stomachs. After that the training wheels come off, and we balance our food the way God intended…with a thankful heart and not a guilty conscience.

House Call With Rita Hancock, MD

Question: In your book *The Eden Diet* you have a technique that I now use before I eat. It is called the Apple Test. The idea is so simple, but it has changed the way I look at food. How do you explain this test to your patients?

Dr. Rita Hancock : The premise is that when you are physically hungry, you'll eat anything—even an apple. To take the test, do the following. If you crave a particular food, such as cheesecake, imagine it sitting on a plate next to a beautiful, shiny, perfect, bright red apple. Ask yourself, "Am I hungry enough to eat the apple?" If the answer is no, you don't get to eat the cheesecake. You may want the cheesecake, but you're not physically hungry for it.

Let me be clear. I'm not saying that you "should" eat the apple if you "would" eat the apple, or that apples are right to eat and cheesecake is wrong to eat. I'm simply saying that if you wouldn't eat the apple at that point, you are not physically hungry. This technique will work with any food that you consider to be neutral—an item that you don't love or hate. This test is just one way that you can rate our hunger before eating.

Chapter Four

KICKING UP SOME DUST

WHEN I MADE the decision to write this book, my goal was to be truthful about my experiences. I had a definite opinion about exercise when I weighed three hundred pounds. It could be expressed with just one sentence—"Hate it!" I always joked that if you see me out jogging, watch out. It means that I am being chased by an angry bear.

I was often tired and out of breath even without "jogging." I believed at the time that this was a natural part of the aging process. Most people over the age of thirty don't feel like teenagers anymore. As my weight started to climb, my activity level was that of someone twice my age. This wasn't a coincidence. I was carrying the weight of another adult on my back. Even simple things such as climbing the stairs and going to the grocery store felt like a workout.

I knew that if I was ever going to be a healthy weight, exercise had to be a part of the plan. From talking with my doctor and reading countless health magazines, I understood that increasing my physical activity could lower my risk of cardiovascular diseases, diabetes, and cancer. Exercise is that important. So did I go for a two-mile jog on the first day of my weight-loss plan? Nope.

The idea of trying to lower my calories *and* begin an exercise plan at the same time was overwhelming. My faith that I could actually stick with a plan for more than a few days was small. I knew I had to give this whole "lowering my calories" thing a try and make it past the first week. I was honestly like a child trying to take her first steps. I was that shaky.

It wasn't until the middle of May (two months into my weight loss) that I found the courage to get off my couch and move a little bit. After sixty days of watching my portion sizes, I had lost about fifteen pounds. I was feeling my first rush of success. Because I was so obese, no one else had noticed my weight loss. In spite of that, my husband's scale was giving me some good news. Side note: It took several months of getting on the scale every day before it felt like "our scale" rather than "my husband's scale."

My first exercise attempt was a 1.5-mile walk around the city park with my dog. It was a hot, Sunday afternoon, and there were some steep hills to climb. After about fifteen minutes I cheated and cut across the inside of the park. It turned my 1.5-mile walk into something less than one mile.

Did I feel guilty about that? Not at all. When I got back into my car, I glanced in the mirror. My hair was sweaty, my face was red, and I looked like I had run a marathon. What wouldn't have been a big achievement for the average "dog walker" was monumental to me. I had actually done something active, and I knew I was coming back the next day.

There are a few things I learned by this experience that I want you to remember when you start your weight loss:

1. **I didn't begin a diet plan and an exercise plan at the same time.** When I felt strong enough to add exercise, I chose an activity that I found simple and, yes, even enjoyable.

2. **"Getting off the couch" didn't require a lot of expensive equipment or training.**

3. **Progress was gradual.** I added more hills and distance to my walks, but at my own pace. My "less than a mile" eventually became twelve to fifteen

miles per week. Our family dog also lost some belly fat along the way and found a new appreciation for squirrels.

It wasn't until I had lost one hundred pounds that my family celebrated by joining a gym. I'm using the word *celebrate* even though that would have sounded crazy to me just one year before. How can exercise be a celebration? How can it be anything but hard work?

When you've been inactive for a long period of time, it's easy to forget the joy you felt when your body was stronger. Remember playing tag, jumping rope, and catching fireflies as a child? Remember what it felt like when your body had the energy to play on a hot, summer night and keep on playing until you collapsed into bed? You can have a taste of that freedom and strength again, but it all starts with exercise.

This is one area where I believe fear can be our biggest enemy. In elementary school I loved swimming. At three hundred pounds, there was *no way* I was putting on a bathing suit in public. In high school I was on the dance team. At three hundred pounds I was afraid that people would see me and think to themselves, "Look, the dancing hippo from *Fantasia*." In college I took an aerobics class At three hundred pounds, pushing a vacuum cleaner was aerobic!

I understand from experience that when you are overweight, you don't have a lot faith in your body. You may wonder if you will ever have strength and endurance again. The day that I laced up my dusty tennis shoes and drove to the park, my confidence was small, probably about the size of a mustard seed. And like a seed it grew into an honest appreciation for my body's ability to meet my demands and get stronger with each test. The same will be true for you if you find your courage and just start moving.

AN ACTION PLAN FOR YOUR ACTION PLAN

Here is a quick checklist of the things you will need to know before you start exercising.

1. **Talk to your doctor and get the green light to begin an exercise program.** If you are obese, it is pretty common to have knee pain, back pain, hip pain, and the like. The list can be long when your body is carrying around too much weight. Your doctor will ask about your family history and might recommend low-impact activities that "go easy" at first on your aches and pains. In the case of my three-hundred-pound body, losing weight minimized and eventually eliminated my joint pain. I had what I called "bad knees" until my weight dropped to a healthy number. My knees are now pain-free.

2. **Don't implement a new diet and a new exercise plan on the same day.** This is especially true if you have a lot of "dieting practice" in your past. I won't call them diet failures, because they gave you some valuable information about what doesn't work for you. Look at it as practice for the real thing. In my case I had to become confident lowering my daily calories *before* adding exercise to my plan.

3. **Don't spend a lot of money in the beginning.** When you get excited about starting an exercise plan, you may have the urge to buy expensive equipment or sign a long-term gym contract. *Hang on.* Before you open your wallet, experiment and see what activities you really enjoy. Maybe riding a bike will be your plan for the first six months. Maybe you enjoy music, and a dance class is how you want to

start. We have a tendency to picture "working out" as a treadmill and free weights. Your plan is just that... *your plan*. Make it enjoyable for you.

4. **Make an exercise schedule that fits your life and your energy levels.** When I made my first attempt at fitness, my goal was to walk my dog for one hour at least three or four times a week. I exercised in the evening after dinner because I have more energy at night. That might not be the right schedule for you. Maybe your lunch hour is the best time to squeeze in some exercise. My husband is a morning person and enjoys working out at the crack of dawn. There are a lot of crazy people out there like him. You may be one of them!

5. **Your ultimate goal is to build strength and endurance.** When an activity gets boring or feels too easy, it's time to try new things. Your heart rate can be a good guide for this. Walking up a hill may get your heart pumping when you first start. After several weeks you'll be able to scale that same hill without breaking a sweat. It's a sign that you are getting stronger and need to add some additional activities into your fitness routine.

After about eight months I noticed that walking my dog wasn't getting my heart rate as high as it did in the beginning. I added my son's Wii Fit to my routine and selected the games with yoga, balance, and strength training. Since then I've also added a gym membership for the cardio and resistance machines, free weights, Zumba, and ballroom dance classes. It may be a sign that I have a short attention span, but I like alternating these activities throughout the week. It keeps exercise fun.

Don't forget that your physical activities can give you some breathing room as you try to stay under your daily calorie goal. I love the flexibility of knowing I can "buy" an extra cookie by spending fifteen minutes on a good cardio machine. Your plan will start to feel like a piggy bank. The more active you are, the more calories you can eat and lose weight.

THE POWER OF PLUS-SIZED FITNESS

The Cooper Institute, a nonprofit health organization, studied twenty-two thousand subjects.[1] These participants varied in age from thirty to eighty-three years. The research measured each person's body composition (fat-to-muscle ratio). Both the normal weight and overweight participants were put through treadmill tests. The institute followed these subjects for eight years and began to see a trend that was surprising to physicians and dieticians.

Four hundred twenty-eight of the participants died during the eight years of the study. Individuals who were overweight but fit (as measured by the treadmill tests) were two times less likely to have died than those who were lean but not fit. Even more interesting was this result: the all-cause mortality rate of fit, overweight individuals wasn't significantly different than the fit, lean participants. Fitness, rather than fat, was a better indicator of a person's overall ability to stay alive. Exercise is medicine without a co-pay or nasty list of side effects.

OUR HANG-UPS WITH HANGING SKIN

When I weighed three hundred pounds, I had visions of what I would look like if I were smaller. I dreamed of the clothes I would wear, the roller coasters I could ride, and the airplane seats I wouldn't fill to overflowing. At no time during these fantasies did I wonder, "Gee, where is all this extra skin going to go when I lose weight?" It was a kind older lady (a waitress in a Tex-Mex restaurant of all places) who told me I better start exercising if I didn't want my skin to hang like the fabric on a curtain rod. Oh, how the truth can sting with a side of salsa!

Exercise must become a part of your plan if your goal is a life-long "healthier ever after." Exercise is also important if your goal is "toned ever after." So let's have an honest conversation about the wiggly, jiggly, loose skin we all dread after weight loss. After my conversation with the well-meaning waitress, I wondered if my skin would resemble a shar-pei if I lost 155 pounds. Could it ever "bounce back" after so many years of obesity? How many thousands of sit-ups would it take? I didn't have high hopes.

After more than three years of regular exercise, I have some good news to report from this forty-year-old body of mine. Do I still have some extra skin? Yes. Does it bother me? It is only an issue if I'm wearing a miniskirt, and I'm too "mature" to pull that off anyway. Has it improved with exercise? Absolutely!

With a good combination of stretching, aerobic, and strength-training exercises, your body can replace some of the space currently occupied by fat with more muscle. I've had a lot of luck with resistance machines. When you walk into a gym, these are the machines with a weight stack and pulley system that give you resistance against a fixed movement. They can help you tone and tighten the muscles underneath sagging skin. This, in turn, can actually tighten the skin. Don't be intimated by these machines. They are great for beginners!

I went into the world of fitness like most people who learned about exercise from watching and not doing. I was badly informed. I thought crunches would get rid of belly fat and leg lifts would remove my "saddle bags." After several months of frustration and a few helpful words from a certified athletic trainer, I finally learned the golden rule of fitness. *You can't target fat loss in a specific part of your body with exercise.*

Don't panic! You will lose fat if you consistently burn more calories than you eat, but it can't be targeted. During my weight loss I lost fat in some very strange places. My feet got smaller. My ring size went from a 9 to a 5, and I don't even want to talk about my changing bra size. I wasn't able to avoid fat loss in one area and target fat loss in another, but I did target muscle development in my abdominals, legs, and arms.

There is more good news. With a regular strength-training program, you can reduce your *overall* body fat and increase your lean muscle mass to burn calories more efficiently. As you gain muscle, your body has a bigger "engine" to burn calories more efficiently, which can result in weight loss. The more toned your muscles, the easier it is to control your weight. It needs to be a part of your plan!

The Whole Truth—So Help Me God

There are still days when I would rather sit on my couch than get up and move. Sad, but true. When the weather is too hot, too cold, or too wet, it can be easy to come up with an excuse not to exercise. That is when it's time for some mental negotiations.

Agree in your mind to exercise, but go with half of the time or distance you had originally planned. Once you have your tennis shoes on and your heart is pumping, who knows what will happen? Endorphins are real and can be a great boost to "keep going" once you get started. Over time, getting even a small amount of daily exercise can add up to a lot of lost pounds. When I finish a walk or a trip to the gym, I am always glad I made the effort. Remember that feeling when you are in "negotiations" with your brain.

House Call With Nick Yphantides, MD

Question: I'm going to play the devil's advocate on the subject of exercise because these are the excuses that I had to remain sedentary. Give me your response.

"Dr. Nick, I would work out, but there is something good on television."

Dr. Yphantides: You can record the show for viewing later. Most cable systems and satellite providers have this option, or just use an old VCR player. I personally limit my TV watching to news and sports and love to watch while on a stationary bike, treadmill, or StairMaster. It's a perfect distraction and an ideal way to combine something enjoyable with something healthy. I'd rather live a sitcom or a captivating reality show than watch one.

Question: "Dr. Nick, I can't get a babysitter."

Dr. Yphantides: Most fitness centers offer some sort of child-care program. You can also offer to watch your friend's children in exchange for watching yours while you exercise. Take your kids on a walk with you. Model healthy behavior early in life!

Question: "Dr. Nick, it hurts my knees to walk on a treadmill."

Dr. Yphantides: Then ride a recumbent bike or swim. When your knees get used to physical activity after years without use, you can try walking on a treadmill again. As you lose weight, the pain will decrease and your capacity will be enhanced!

Question: "But Dr. Nick, you don't know what it's like to be the fattest person in the gym."

Dr. Yphantides: Ah, I caught you. Yes, I do know what it is like. But excuses are excuses, and the mind has an amazing ability to rationalize and create excuses to get you out of the things you don't want to do. My advice is that when an excuse comes to mind, you immediately think of something else. Your life may depend on it. Gyms, especially community gyms, can be a very safe and accepting place.

Nick Yphantides, MD is the chief medical officer for San Diego county. In March of 2001 this 467-pound doctor embarked on an ambitious yet creative weight-loss program by taking a "radical sabbatical." He crisscrossed the country with family and friends and attended more than one hundred major-league baseball games on a plan that included exercise and two or three protein shakes a day. By the end of the baseball season that fall, 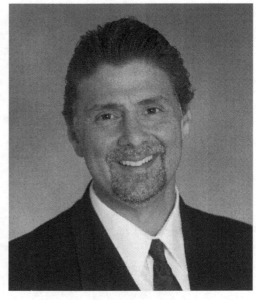 Dr. Yphantides came home weighing 249 pounds. He continued to work toward his final goal weight by watching his calories, eating smaller portions, and exercising. In the summer of 2002 Dr. Yphantides weighed 197 pounds. He went on to write the book My Big Fat Greek Diet to tell his story and share the seven pillars of weight loss that he shares with anyone looking to improve their health and fitness level.

Chapter Five

SILENCING THE LIES

URING THE LAST few years I've had the opportunity to travel and speak with groups about healthy weight loss. I admit that my primary focus was generally on those in the audience who would be categorized as obese. They reminded me of me. I knew these were "my" people—*very* overweight individuals who understand what it is really like to struggle with food. Whew, was I wrong!

Over and over again I was shocked to see the one-hundred-sixty-pound lady in my audience just as upset and desperate to find solutions as the three-hundred-pound lady. I remember thinking, "What is your deal? You are crying over ten or fifteen extra pounds? Are you serious?" Needless to say, I had some learning to do about food and its complicated relationship with our stomachs and our brains.

The one-hundred-sixty-pound woman could be at a healthy weight in just a few weeks where the three-hundred-pound woman is facing months of work. The one-hundred-sixty-pound woman can shop anywhere she wants while the three-hundred-pound woman is thanking God that the one store in town with plus-size clothing now has a size 28. The one-hundred-sixty-pound woman doesn't have diabetes or high blood pressure. The three-hundred-pound woman has both. What could these women have in common?

The lies. They have the lies in common.

I have some big "untruths" from my own weight-loss struggles. I've also added a few more from those I've had the opportunity to meet and mentor. It doesn't seem to matter how many diets you've been on. It doesn't matter how much weight you need to lose. At our very core, we are all flawed. We are willing to believe the worst about our character when we are weak. We question why God would bother to love us at all. These lies can bring us to our knees in hopelessness if left to run wild in our minds. Are any of these big lies hiding in the small corners of your brain?

TEN BIG WHOPPERS (LIES NOT THE CANDY)

1. I'm just too busy to spend time exercising or cooking healthy food.

2. It is selfish to focus my time on getting healthy. My family would feel abandoned.

3. Trying to lose weight is pointless. When has it ever worked before?

4. Obesity runs in my family. It's just the way we are, and I will always be fat.

5. "Skinny" people have more self-control and discipline than I have.

6. If I cut back on the foods I love, my life is going to be miserable.

7. My size isn't really that unhealthy. I look good carrying extra pounds, and it doesn't bother me at all. (This is also called "my man likes my curves!")

8. I'm on medication that makes it hard for me to lose weight. I also have bad knees, a bad back, bad feet, and more.

9. I work hard, and now it's time to celebrate. I deserve a little treat.

10. I can't live forever, so eat, drink, and be merry.

Read this list, and read it again. The statements above may be as comfortable to you as an old pair of shoes. Maybe you've lived with them as constant companions for years. My big lies were three, six, and nine on the list. And just like an old pair of shoes they gave me no support and had a definite stink when I examined them too closely.

Recognize these lies for what they are. If you've struggled with food in the past, I guarantee that these comfortable, old lies will come out of the closet on the very day you start to watch your calories or begin an exercise plan. They may be different than my Ten Big Whoppers, but I'm guessing that they are just as deadly.

Before you begin this weight-loss plan, take the time to write your own "whoppers." Grab a piece of paper or use the journaling feature on our online calorie tracker. If you've lived with the lies as long as I did, it will be easy. The toughest part might be the next step: writing down what you know is the truth. It's amazing, but your lies won't stand a chance against the bright light of honesty. Don't be afraid to turn on that light! Below are ten truths from my own journal.

Ten Truths (From Someone Who Has Been There)

1. I will take a hard look at my schedule and find the time to take care of myself.

2. I will set a positive example for my family and be a living lesson of faith.

3. I've learned from my past weight-loss attempts. I now have valuable information to move forward.

4. My genetics will not be an excuse for bad choices.

5. I want more than just willpower for this journey. Through faith I have God's power and the strength of those who love me.

6. I can eat and enjoy foods in every color of the rainbow...not just beige, brown, and white.

7. By losing weight, I will lower my risk for diabetes, cancer, and heart disease.

8. My doctor is an active partner in my weight loss. Together we will find solutions that fit my individual needs.

9. I work hard, and I am wonderfully made. Today I will make healthy choices that make my body stronger and let the Lord hold tomorrow.

10. I have a limited amount of time on this earth, and God has a plan for my life that requires the best that I can give Him.

Something powerful happens when you see the truth for your life written down. It becomes more than just wishful thinking. It is pure honesty in black and white. It can defeat the lies.

GETTING HEALTHY BY GETTING OVER YOURSELF

I have some good news for all of the perfectionists in the crowd. No one spends hours thinking about your size. You aren't being judged as harshly as you might imagine, and the people who love you see more than your weight. We are each a unique and crazy mix of talent, humor, generosity, faith, compassion, and perseverance.

Perfectionists can lose sight of this. I thought everyone labeled me as "lazy and undisciplined" when I weighed three hundred pounds. That may sound self-deprecating, but it was really pride. I thought about my weight constantly, and I assumed that the world had nothing better to do than join me. I had to get over myself. When the people around us really "know" us, they see a complex package that is more than just the wrapping on the outside.

First impressions are tough on the obese. And if that obese person is also a perfectionist, meeting new people can be downright painful. Humans are wired to pick up hundreds of tiny details about the stranger standing in front of us. Size and shape are two of the many "scales" we use to evaluate a person's appearance, health, and yes, even a person's character. Obese perfectionists are all too aware that the world makes unfair assumptions about their discipline and work ethic.

The link between perfectionism and addiction is well documented. It's ironic that our culture uses phrases such as "he let himself go" and "she stopped caring about herself" to describe someone who is overweight. The opposite is often the case. Obesity can be the result of a bar that is set impossibly high. When the perfectionist fails to clear the bar, an addiction can dull the pain of failure and provide some brief comfort. In the case of a food addiction, high-fat/high-sugar foods trigger the pleasure center in the brain It's a serotonin "warm hug" to the rescue!

I've decided (apprentice philosopher that I am) that so much of our life can be defined by how we respond to struggles. Optimists may call these struggles "challenging," but the rest of us simply call them "stressful." They are the tough situations we face every day, and they generally fall within five categories: work stress, financial pressures, health problems/fatigue, conflicts with relationships, and bad weather/natural disasters.

When faced with a problem, we each create a picture in our minds of the solution. How can I fix this? Will I suffer? What will victory look like? I believe the details of this mental picture set us up either for failure or for success. Let's make this simple and use our old friends (the tortoise and the hare) to explore this more.

The tortoise

His stress: Through the holiday season, the tortoise ate too many fruitcakes and ran up some credit card debt (buying Turtle Wax for his lovely wife). It is now January 2, and the tortoise is looking for a solution.

The plan: The tortoise decides to walk to work in order to get more exercise and spend less money on gas. He must leave for work forty minutes early every morning, but he feels that he can handle this small sacrifice. It will take several months to reach his goal.

His temptations: There are several snowy days in late January when the tortoise drives into work. It's just too cold to walk. As a result, the scale doesn't move that week, and he must spend more money on gas.

His response: The tortoise tells his wife that he is disappointed that his journey to lose weight and pay off debt got sidetracked. There is a chance of sleet this morning, but he is determined to get back on the plan. His wife gives him four warm boots to wear, and the tortoise starts walking to work.

The hare

His stress: Like the tortoise, the hare gained weight during the Christmas season eating too much carrot cake. He also ran up some credit card debt (buying hare hair care products for his lovely wife).

The plan: Restrict his calorie intake by eating nothing but lettuce and run to work every morning. Because of his natural speed, the hare doesn't see the need to leave early for work. He'll just sprint. (Perfectionist warning: pride. Although perfectionism and addiction are generally indicators of low self-esteem, these individuals can also have attitudes of grandiosity. Perfectionists think they should be able to outrun ordinary mortals.) The hare is on a mission to lose twenty pounds and pay off his credit card debt within one month. (Perfectionist warning: setting unrealistic goals.)

His struggle: After the first week the hare was able to lose three pounds and save $12.52 in gas. It's progress, but it seems too slow to the hare. (Perfectionist warning: a mistrust of success when it happens. If a perfectionist happens to actually achieve a goal, he/she doesn't think, "Yes, I'm getting somewhere!" Perfectionists conclude that the bar is set too low.)

His response: The hare is embarrassed to share his "small" victory with this wife. (Perfectionist warning: a need to go it alone. These individuals see the need for support as a weakness.) After losing only two pounds the next week, the hare decides that his plan is a failure. He feels hungry, tired, and disappointed. If he can't lose five pounds a week, he must be a loser. (Perfectionist warning: harsh punishment for setbacks. After losing confidence, the plan is abandoned.) The next morning the hare has a slice of carrot cake for breakfast and drives to work.

The end to this story hasn't changed since your childhood. Slow and steady won the race. It's the age-old power of incremental progress. The tortoise was able to slim down and pay off his credit card debt through a plan that required patience. His journey also required an ability to forgive himself when he got off track and the humility to ask for help when he needed it.

As a "hare" in recovery I understand that perfectionism is generally rooted in fear. We greatly exaggerate how the world will respond if we fail. It's as if our internal "if/then" statements are on steroids. "If I can't lose twenty pounds in one month, then my family will abandon me, the world economy will collapse, and my dog won't come when called."

I learned after twenty years of abandoned weight-loss attempts that I might be big, but I'm not that big of a deal. People are fighting their own challenges and don't spend hours dissecting mine. They have better things to do. In fact, being honest about our imperfections takes the pressure off of everyone else and makes for much better stories at dinner parties.

It might be hard to image this today, but your slow and imperfect steps toward a healthy weight could inspire someone who feels hopeless about their own obesity. The best lessons start with the words, "OK, here is where I made my mistakes..." The ways you coped with stress, handled temptations, and reached out for help can teach in ways that a "perfect march" toward a healthy weight never could.

When we are in the heat of a struggle, it's tough to believe that the Lord can make something good come out of our pain. He can. Take a deep breath and let Jesus be the perfect one.

LIES INTO LIGHT

To battle the whoppers that will be coming your way, you will need the ultimate lie detector. When you feel tempted, you will need a strength that goes beyond your own. When you feel discouraged, you will need a loving Father and the unshakable foundation that faith and prayer can provide. It can be a base of support that will stand strong even when the people in your life disappoint you.

Even before day one of your weight loss, it is important to have realistic expectations about the people in your life. Don't be surprised or crushed when those who love you let you down. It's going to happen from time to time. We're going to talk in the next chapter about what to look for when you are building your support team, but understand that even the best "cheerleader" can't meet *all* of your physical and emotional needs during your weight loss. That is a position only God can fill. I'd like to explore this more, but first, a few disclaimers.

I don't have a degree in theology, and I'm not an ordained minister. I get nervous praying out loud in front of other people, and sometimes I struggle finding Philemon in the Bible. It is a short book!

So what *do* I know about God? All the good stuff!

1. He sees what is possible.

2. He can make it happen when we have faith.

3. His ways are higher than our ways.

It is not the Lord's will for any of us to waste the precious hours of our lives as a slave to our appetite. Maybe you have a lot of plans for your life, but understand this: God had plans for your life *before you were born*. You will receive strength that will be impossible to measure when you ask God to make His will your will.

That is the all-important step I took in March of 2007. That's it! I had to admit that my plan would never be enough on its own. I might understand the science of calories and exercise, but I didn't have the willpower to turn all that knowledge into success. My vision was worthless, because I couldn't fight the years of anger and the despair alone. In the darkness I cried out to the Lord and gave it all away.

My "this is enough" moment was just that easy, and it was just that hard. I want to be very clear about what happened that day. I didn't pray and ask God to *help* me. I had tried that little trick for twenty years, and it was just my lame attempt to stay in control. I didn't give God a trial run at leading my life. This wasn't going to be a case of, "You can have my life, God. At least until I want it back." I'm telling you that I prayed and got out of the way.

Once you take that huge step, you might wonder how it works here on the ground. Do I feel weaker now that I've given up all that control? Do I have to ask for God's permission before every bite of food? That's what I would have guessed when I weighed three hundred pounds. I believed that if I let God lead, I would be forced to live on a diet of celery, unleavened bread, and ice chips. I pictured myself weeping in front of doughnut cases while lashing my back with licorice whips. I was going to be a pitiful, wretched sight.

We know we have a perfect Lord. So why are we so surprised when His will for our life is perfect? With God in control, food is no longer my enemy. I eat meat, potatoes, bread, lots of fruits and vegetables, and even desserts. I enjoy hamburgers, pizza, pasta, and ice cream. I've enjoyed all of these things since day one of my weight loss. I eat delicious foods in the right amounts. And when it's time to walk away from the table, I walk away. All that former anger has been replaced with an almost indescribable feeling of freedom.

I don't know how long it's been since you've thought about your relationship with God or took the time to pray. I don't know if you opened this book today with a strong faith in the Lord or a faith as small as a mustard seed. God has a plan for your life either way. Are you curious what it might be? Take a little time today and ask Him.

The Whole Truth—So Help Me God

I wish I could tell you that the lies will go away forever once you confront them with the truth. That hasn't happened for me. I have moments when I remember those old, stinky shoes with fondness, and sometimes I try them on again for size. I make unhealthy choices and have a "bad" day from time to time. I eat too many cookies or skip the gym because it is raining outside. I'll tell myself that I've worked hard and "deserve a break." It's OK. Although the lies may never go away while we walk on this earth, they will grow weaker every time we honestly confront them for what they are. Lies. Don't allow them to turn a bad day into a bad week into a bad month. Pray and let God shine the light of truth on them!

House Call With Rita Hancock, MD

Question: What do you recommend to your patients who struggle with emotional eating?

Dr. Hancock: I direct them to a free download I created on my website www.TheEdenDiet.com. I'll tell you about it here, but you can also download it by clicking on the blinking "Break Free" button at the bottom right of the home page.

I found with my own history of emotional eating that these steps can help us determine why we want to eat when we aren't truly hungry.

1. Find a nice, quiet place, where you can have private time with God.

2. Notice that you're feeling "emotional," and take the main emotion that is bothering you "captive" in your mind.

3. Name your emotion. Is it fear, anger, sadness, or anxiety?

4. Accept yourself in spite of how you feel because that's what God does. In fact, emphatically remind yourself of this, saying it out loud, over and over again. "It's OK for me to feel [fill in the blank]. I accept myself fully, just as God accepts me fully." The spoken word is a powerful thing, especially when it lines up with the Word of God.

5. While focusing on God in prayer, directly experience the negative emotion in His presence. Even if it feels uncomfortable to do this, remember that the emotion itself won't actually kill you.

6. Choose another activity besides eating if you feel the urge to "do" something with the emotion. Perhaps you can exercise or take care of something you've been procrastinating about.

7. Thank God for the revelation that it's OK to feel negative emotions. It doesn't make you a bad person. Thank Him profusely. Out loud.

8. Forgive yourself if you believe you've done something wrong (to create these emotions), and

forgive others whose actions might have led to those emotions. State your forgiveness out loud.

9. Prayerfully come to the point where you're willing to separate yourself from those thoughts and emotions. Thank God for allowing you to psychologically separate from those issues. Tell Him out loud, "Thank You, God, for allowing me to separate from this problem so I can move on with my life." Say it like you mean it, and say it over and over again if need be.

10. Find something better to think about than the thoughts that led to those emotions. Focus on positive thoughts. Then you can more easily feel the fruit of the Spirit.

11. Breathe. As you deal with these emotions, take deep breaths occasionally. As you exhale, literally breathe out your stress and let your physical body relax.

Question: I've met so many people who struggle with obesity. Many feel a strong burden to take care of others and not "let anyone down." Does this attitude make weight loss more difficult?

Dr. Hancock: I believe it can. But a long time ago I learned that I don't necessarily have to do everything that others want or expect me to do. It's not possible to please everybody all the time. I also learned that I'm not necessarily even supposed to try to please everybody. Sometimes others' expectations of me are downright unfair or irrational.

Realizing these things took a lot of pressure off of me. God didn't necessarily create me to do all the good things that I could be doing with my time or to rescue everybody who wants my time or my help. God created me because He loves me. I'm His beloved child, not a "tool." He loves me just as much as He loves the people He wants me to help.

I can't even begin to tell you how much peace I feel knowing that I don't have to "do" to be good enough for God. I would ask any person who feels this pressure: How about you? Do you feel like you're nothing more than a tool? Do you feel anxious when you're not involved in a do-good project? If so, maybe your overextended schedule and resultant anxiety are leading you to stress eat. Maybe your anxiety even manifests as physical illness or pain through the mind-body-spirit connection.

If I just described you, hear me now: you are not just a tool. You are God's beloved child—fearfully and wonderfully (though imperfectly) made, just like me. Rest in that scriptural truth rather than in a box of HoHos the next time you feel compelled to take on another good but unnecessary, time-consuming project that stresses you out.

Chapter Six

BUILDING SUPPORT ON A BUDGET

I HAVE NO IDEA where in the world you are right now. I don't know if you have a spouse, children, extended family, or friends. I am willing to go out on a limb and guess that you are not living alone on a deserted island. That is good news for you! It's time to get the people around you ready for your weight-loss journey. It's time for some honesty. It's time for a little bit of confession.

THE DANGERS OF PRIDE

Depending on your individual personality, this could be the hardest step in the entire book for you to take. Remember the hare in the last chapter? If someone in early 2007 had told me to "'fess up" about my weight-loss struggles, I would have grabbed one of my Big Whoppers and let it fly. My favorite was always, "Trying to lose weight is pointless. I'll just fail again. Why bother to announce it to the world?" It was easier for me to laughingly admit defeat to my family and friends than risk the embarrassment of still having hope.

Underneath it all this wasn't Linda being humble about her weight. It was the opposite. Along with all of the fat I was also obese on pride. I could point to a wonderful husband, bright and beautiful children, good friends, and a rewarding job. So many things in my life could be defined as a success. It was my own vanity that craved for people to pay attention to everything that was healthy in my life and ignore the unhealthy.

From where I stood, it seemed plain silly to shine a harsh light on my weaknesses. What if my family and friends judged me? What if they start paying more attention to the food I ate? What if I'm not able to lose the weight? Will they decide that I'm just too disgusting to be around? These fears, of course, didn't have much to do with reality. It's not like my obesity was a secret. When I weighed three hundred pounds, an absolute stranger could have guessed that I struggled with overeating.

Your issues with food may be easier to hide than mine were. Maybe your family has no idea how many hours you spend focused on your weight. Maybe your friends only see the "in control" person you show to the world. But if the idea of confessing your struggles makes you break out in a cold sweat, maybe it's time to put your pride on a diet.

Admitting my two-decade struggle with food was so hard for me that I didn't do it during the early days of my weight loss. This is a situation where I'm asking you to "do what I say and not what I did." I foolishly avoided this step up in 2007. I think God must have carried me because I didn't have anywhere else to draw support.

From experience you probably understand that the first weeks of a new diet plan are fragile. I tried to walk on those fragile legs without any help on the ground. I didn't tell anyone that I was trying to lose weight. What if it didn't work? I quietly lowered my calories, measured my portions, and fought my cravings—alone and miserable.

I can't prove this scientifically, but I have a theory about high-calorie foods. When you want to avoid them, these treats will tease you, taunt you, and chase you like a bully around every corner. Doughnuts will appear on your desk at work. The cheap guy at the office will offer to buy ice cream for the entire staff. Everyone you know will have a birthday and refuse to celebrate without you. My first week of weight loss I barely survived the chase. I was so tired.

My husband was the first to notice I was miserable. Actually, he noticed I was crabby. I explained in a calm voice (or more likely whined in a shrill voice) that I was trying to lose weight by low-ering my calories. I confessed that the last week had been "really hard." He looked at me and immediately said, "Great. I'll do it with you."

That was it. No laughing, no eye rolling, no sarcastic "better luck this time." Instant support. It was the knowledge I could talk about my temptations and setbacks. It was a pledge that when I was weak, he would be strong. I realized I could have had this strong foundation from day one if I would have asked for it.

The people who know you and love you can be a blessing during your weight loss if you honestly tell them about your struggles. Be specific about the reasons you want to lose weight: diabetes in the family, high blood pressure, risk of cancer, running out of places to buy clothes, or even can't fit on a roller coaster. It is important that your family and friends realize that your desire to lose weight goes beyond vanity.

My primary support is my spouse, but yours doesn't have to be. He/she may not be the right fit for you. That's OK. A lack of enthu-siasm from your spouse isn't an excuse to stay unhealthy. Let's say it again. Do not let an uninvolved or negative attitude in your home rob you of the life God has planned for you. Quietly lead by example (without nagging) and see how the Lord uses your faith.

In a very real sense you are creating a team that will stay with you through every "scale is stuck" moment. You must choose your support players wisely and give them very specific information on how they can help you win. We're going to examine in a little more detail what to look for when creating your foundation and specifi-cally what these important people can do to support you.

APPROACH WEIGHT-LOSS CONTESTS WITH CAUTION

When your family, friends, and coworkers hear about your upcoming weight-loss plan, they may recommend a little compe-tition to help you get started. Come on, how can you get more supportive than that? Not only will they hear about your struggles, but also these caring souls will literally feel your pain! Plus, you will have the chance to win cash or a wonderful showcase of prizes. What's not to like? There is actually quite a bit *not* to like if your goal is long-term success.

Please understand I'm not trying to take away anyone's idea of "fun" weight loss. And as you read this section, I'm sure you'll remember one or two lucky people who lost pounds during a weight-loss contest and actually kept it off. Please don't write and tell me about your old college roommate who lost more weight than any other girl in your dorm and won one hundred dollars. I'm sure she hasn't gained a single pound back since you ran this diet contest during the Clinton administration. We're going to look past the exceptions, and take a hard look at the 99.99 percent of us who need this rule.

Can you kick off your diet with a contest? Absolutely. Will your competitive spirit help you lose weight? Possibly. Will you walk away from the contest with a healthy attitude about food and exercise and a plan that will last for a lifetime? Probably not. Contests (by their very nature) can encourage some unhealthy patterns of eating and exercise.

1. It is all about eating fewer calories than the competition.

Too often nutrition is left in the ditch as you run toward your "weigh-in" every week. I have friends who dropped their daily calories well below 1,000 in order to win a contest. This isn't a pattern of eating that you can sustain over the long haul and for good reason. You're hungry. Your body isn't getting what it needs to thrive.

2. Exercise feels like torture.

Weight-loss contests can hijack your exercise plan by taking away the important element of patience. An eager dieter attempts to go from coach potato to Olympic athlete in just one day. Gone is the advantage of building strength and endurance over time. It becomes an attitude of "I'm going to win this competition and work out constantly!" Also gone is any concept of fun. It becomes all about burning more calories than the competition. Very few people will want to continue this exercise schedule after the weight-loss competition has ended because they feel battered and bruised.

I know from experience that starting a new exercise plan also requires energy. If your daily calorie intake is too low (because food has become the enemy), it will be hard to get up and get moving. Putting your body through a new exercise plan on an empty stomach will be something close to torture. You'll be looking at the longest two and a half hours of your week! Gone is the element of fueling your exercise with the right amount of calories. You'll walk away from the weight-loss competition with a false belief that exercise leaves you tired. Over time the opposite is true. Don't believe me? Pay attention to the exercise veterans you see walking out of a gym, fitness center, and dance studio. You might witness some sweat but probably no tears.

3. Your success isn't "good" enough.

This is perhaps the most damaging attitude that can come out of a weight-loss competition. Too often I've seen people put their hearts into losing weight and walk away disappointed because they "lost only two pounds this week." They miss out on the feeling of accomplishment that should come from moving in the right direction. It's all about losing more than the other guy. A two-pound drop was a *good* week for me during my weight loss. I'd step off the scale and yell, "Yes!" Anything that takes away that joy is a bad idea.

So if weight-loss competitions are off limits, can those around you still play an active role in your journey? Absolutely. The rest of this chapter is dedicated to putting those who love you to work on your behalf!

CLIP THE WINGS OF YOUR "FOOD ANGELS"

These wonderful cooks can be anywhere—at church, at work, in your neighborhood, or in your house. They whip up amazing treats and leave them on your desk, on your front porch, and next to your La-Z-Boy chair. They can also turn into "food devils" and make you feel guilty if you don't try one, two, or five!

This is another group you must speak with *before* starting a weight-loss plan. They can be a blessing if you give them guidance, and they can be a curse if you don't get them on your team. Your conversation with a food angel might go something like this: "You are such a great cook, and I love everything you make. I've struggled with my weight for a long time, and it's hard for me to stop with just one of your cookies, cupcakes, and casseroles. I'm going to need your help with this."

Many of the food angels in my life actually became a part of my weight-loss success. Because of their talents in the kitchen, they created delicious recipes that were lower in calories and fat. These people generally want to feed those around them as an expression of love. Nothing will make them happier than watching you eat their new, healthier recipes.

With any homemade dish, even those proclaiming to be low-calorie, portion sizes will be important. My favorite "diet" brownies can still pack a calorie punch if I eat four servings. That may sound like common sense, but we have a tendency to be a little too relaxed when we hear those magical words "low fat and low calorie." Explain this to your food angels, and enlist their help in controlling portion sizes.

WHAT MOVES YOU?

Do you know the answer to that question? Beyond preparing lower calorie dishes, how can those who care about you show support in a way that *truly* motivates you? This is a subject that will be very important when you talk with your family and friends about your upcoming weight loss and the goals/rewards you would like to set.

Dr. Gary Chapman has a set of books that I would like to recommend. In *The Five Love Languages* Dr. Chapman goes into wonderful detail on what motivates us and makes us feel loved. Before you begin recruiting your support team, go online and read more at http://www.5lovelanguages.com/assessments or purchase one of his love languages books. To get you started, there is a short quiz that can help you determine which of the languages you "speak." Dr. Chapman found that most men and women are motivated in one of five ways:[1]

1. Words of affirmation

Actions don't always speak louder than words. If this is your language, unsolicited compliments mean the world to you. Hearing the words such as "I love you," "you look great," and "good job" are important—hearing the reasons behind that love sends your spirits skyward. Insults can leave you shattered and are not easily forgotten.

If words of affirmation is your language, tell your friends and family how motivating their comments can be. During my weight loss, positive feedback was a tremendous boost. If I looked even one pound lighter, I wanted to hear about it. I didn't want to be told lies, but I welcomed even the smallest truth!

2. Quality time

In the vernacular of quality time, nothing says "I love you" like full, undivided attention. Being there for this type of person is critical, but really being there—with the TV off, fork and knife down, and all chores and tasks on standby—makes this person feel truly special and loved. Dr. Chapman has found that distractions, postponed dates, or the failure to listen can be especially hurtful for this group.

If quality time is your language, explain to your friends and family how important their undivided attention will be for you. Ask for face-to-face accountability and support from them without distractions. This might require hiring a baby sitter, taking the phone off the hook, or even hiding the remote control!

3. Receiving gifts

Don't mistake this for materialism. The receiver of gifts thrives on the love, thoughtfulness, and effort behind the gift. If you speak this language, the perfect gift or gesture shows that you are known, you are cared for, and you are prized above whatever was sacrificed to bring the gift to you.

If receiving gifts is your language, setting up rewards during your weight loss will be important and also a lot of fun. Ask for help from your family and friends to determine small, incentive gifts that can be given to you during each milestone of your plan. And to make things exciting, establish a "grand prize" that you will receive when you hit your final weight-loss goal. Be creative! This doesn't have to cost a lot of money, but it will keep your support group involved in your progress. It will also be a wonderful motivation for you.

4. Acts of service

Can taking out the trash be an expression of appreciation? Absolutely! Anything you do to ease the burden of responsibilities weighing on an "acts of service" person will speak volumes. The words he or she most wants to hear: "Let me do that for you." According to Dr. Chapman, laziness, broken commitments, and making more work for them tell speakers of this language their feelings don't matter.

If acts of service is your language, your friends and family can support you with little gestures that won't cost anything but a little bit of their time. Got a chore at home or at work that you'd like to take off your list? Make it a part of your incentive plan. Maybe your support group can empty your trash for a week when you reach your first weight-loss milestone or handle your big "spring cleaning" when you reach your final goal.

5. Physical touch

This language isn't all about the bedroom. A person whose primary language is physical touch is, not surprisingly, very touchy. Hugs, pats on the back, holding hands, and thoughtful touches on the arm, shoulder, or face—they can all be ways to show excitement, concern, care, and love. Physical presence and accessibility are crucial, while neglect or abuse can be unforgivable and destructive.

If physical touch is your language, let your family and friends know how much a hug or a pat on the back will mean to you. There is nothing more precious to me than the monster hug my youngest son gave to me when I reached my weight-loss milestone. His arms could actually wrap around my entire body for the first time. That was the perfect way to celebrate my smaller size and encourage me to keep the weight off.

WHO SHOULD MOVE YOU?

Now that you have some ideas on *what* can motivate you, it's time to decide *who* should motivate you. This might be as easy as talking to a couple of friends who have stood by your side for years. It's a great place to start, but it doesn't have to be your only source of support. There are some things I discovered through trial and error that can help you build your weight-loss cheering section.

1. Contact

Although there is nothing wrong with discussing your weight-loss goals with someone you see only once a year, that won't provide you with enough "on the ground" support. You need the accountability and frequent encouragement that comes from face-to-face contact. Select friends or family who see you *at least* two or three times a month. We are looking for individuals whom you can't hide from when you are struggling.

2. Success

Do you have a friend who battled an addiction and came out healthy on the other side? It doesn't have to be a weight-loss struggle. Some of my best words of encouragement came from former smokers. They understood how powerful cravings and temptations can be. They understood how hard it was for me to try again after years of failure. And because of their victories, they believed I could be victorious too. God must bless these walking "success stories" with a higher level of patience, compassion, and faith. Put these friends on your team!

3. Maturity

This can sometimes come with age but not always. You can probably think of a few "elders" who would rather break a hip than give someone a kind word. They are generally the exception and not the rule. During my weight loss, the seniors in my life were some of my best cheerleaders. These were men and women who weren't afraid to ask about my progress, were happy to share their own stories, and weren't threatened by another person's success. They were quick to tell me that they loved me at any size but applauded every pound that fell. Seniors were an encouraging army of supporters I never expected. You might be surprised who is quietly wishing the best for you through a pair of bifocal glasses.

4. Faith

People generally fall into three categories when it comes to faith and prayer: no faith, a pretend faith, and the real deal. It is my opinion that those with a pretend faith are just as worthless to you (in the area of prayer) as those who admit to having none. Have you ever had someone say that they would pray for you and you just wanted to roll your eyes? You knew that "I'll be praying for you" was just an excuse to get out of a difficult conversation. A more honest comment from that person would have been, "Wow, your situation is really a bummer, but I've got a lot going on in my own life. I have no intention of actually praying for you, but I need to say something to shut you up and make you think I care."

If you are going to take a leap of courage and actually confess your weight-loss struggles to another person, search for individuals who deserve that honor. Does this person remember your birthday, check in on you when you are sick, and care about what is going on in your life? I think we all have friendships that feel a little one-sided. That is generally not a problem if you are planning a quick shopping trip together, but weight loss is an entirely different journey. You need people who live their faith every day and make no apologies. You want strong stuff!

Once you have friends who are committed to pray for you, you want to give them as much power as possible. This isn't the time to be vague or too general. It's important to go beyond saying, "I'm trying to lose weight. Will you pray for me?" Give these people *specific* things to pray for. "It's Thanksgiving, and this has always been a hard time of the year for me. Please pray and ask for God to give me strength. I want to enjoy the holiday, eat delicious foods, and make healthy choices. I need wisdom."

5. Experts

If you've had a primary care physician for any length of time, the subject of weight loss has probably come up. Doctors can be pesky on this subject! They understand how obesity can trigger a whole host of debilitating and deadly diseases. It's not hard to find a physician who is willing to tell you to lose some weight, but you will need more than just a statement of the obvious from your doctor.

Part of your weight-loss foundation will be to evaluate your health care provider with the same attention to detail that I hope he/she is giving to you. Ask yourself these questions:

1. Have you been seeing the same doctor for more than two years?

2. Has the subject of weight loss come up in your examinations?

3. If yes, did he/she make eye contact with you during the discussion and ask you specific questions about your diet, exercise, and lifestyle?

4. Has your doctor given you specific information about calories and nutrition?

5. Would your doctor recognize you on the street and remember your name?

If your health care up to this point has been a series of drop-in clinics or emergency room visits, it's time to establish a long-term relationship with a physician in your area. You want a doctor on your team who can understand the weight-loss struggles in your past, give you a thorough physical today, and become a source of support and information in the future. Be picky. This is important!

The men and women who work in emergency rooms and "after hours" clinics can be outstanding health care providers, but you want your weight-loss support to be more than just a series of first dates. This will be a marriage of sorts between you and your doctor. Have you ever noticed that it is much harder to hide your struggles in a committed relationship? You want that level of trust between you and your physician.

A CASE OF TOUGH LOVE OR TOUGH LUCK FROM YOUR DOC?

"I want to lose weight so that my doctor will respect me and give me better care." This is a motivation for dieting that never occurred to me when I weighed three hundred pounds. Even as my waistline grew a little bigger every year, my doctor continued to provide outstanding care. She gave me constant support and information, having faith that one day I would be ready to lose the weight. If your personal doctor-patient story isn't so positive, you may not be alone.

A study by Johns Hopkins researchers found that physicians often have less respect for obese patients.[2] Doctors were interviewed about their attitudes and gave researchers the honest and ugly truth. According to this study published in the November 2009 issue of the *Journal of General Internal Medicine*, physicians reported that a higher body mass index (BMI) translated into a lower level of respect. In a group of 238 patients, each ten-unit increase in BMI was associated with a 14 percent higher prevalence of low patient respect. The doctors admitted that they made judgments about the character and the intelligence of the people sitting on their examination tables. Those judgments were often based on size.

Despite extensive years of training and multiple degrees on the wall, physicians still look at their patients through human eyes, and they've seen some sad stuff. Doctors have their own "battle" stories: patients who developed diseases, patients who ignored their physicians' advice to lose weight, and patients who died too soon. Doctors never want to be in position where they are fighting harder to keep you alive than you are. A bias against the obese can grow from this frustration.

And while it is fine to understand where this "lack of respect" for the obese originates, tolerating a disrespectful attitude when you are ready to start a weight-loss plan isn't fine. Your doctor's office should be the equivalent of a dieting preschool. It may get messy at times, but it should also be a place of teaching, care, and encouragement.

If your weight-loss journey is like mine, seeing tempting, high-fat foods may make it hard to always follow your doctor's advice. You will make a few bad eating choices (like a preschooler who eats the Elmer's glue). Mistakes will be made. But with some patience for the patient, progress can also be made. You deserve a doctor who understands this and is willing to make an investment of time into your weight-loss education.

I've put together a list to help you see the difference between "tough love" and "tough luck" when it comes to your important doctor-patient relationship. It is the result of asking many people this simple question, "How are things at your doctor's office?" Some of the stories have curled my already frizzy hair.

TOUGH LOVE ON THE EXAMINATION TABLE

1. **Your doctor should bring up the subject of weight.** For those of you who don't want to face your size, this step may sound like torture. Trust me. Take a deep breath and see where the conversation goes. I believe that it is immoral for your primary care physician to avoid discussing the health problems associated with obesity because it makes you uncomfortable. A good doctor is a brave doctor. He or she will risk your wrath in order to save your life.

2. **Your doctor should ask detailed questions.** For someone who was more than one hundred fifty pounds overweight, I was a ninja when it came to avoiding the tough questions. I could stop most weight-loss conversations with this stand-by answer, "Yeah, doc, I know that I need to do something about my weight. I'm going to start a diet and exercise plan right after (insert upcoming holiday here)." A good doctor won't let you end the conversation without more details. He may ask: "What are you eating? When are you eating? Why do you think you are overeating?"

3. **Your doctor should provide you with resources.** Telling you to eat less food and be more

active isn't going to cut it. Primary care physicians are in an ideal place to make weight-loss recommendations that actually work. With so many Americans either overweight or obese, you won't be the first person in your doctor's office asking for dieting advice. Your physician knows from experience what plans can work and what plans are unsafe or promise more than they actually deliver. A good doctor will want to share this information with you and may refer you to a registered dietician or weight-loss center for further support.

A registered dietitian can be a clear head for us in the face of our overwhelming desire to get thin quick. There are certain medical situations where a short-term, rapid approach to weight loss can be lifesaving. For most of us that isn't the case. A registered dietitian can work with your doctor to find a specific menu of foods that fit your specific health and nutrition needs.

During your first visit with a registered dietitian (RD), expect a conversation about your body mass index (BMI). This is the common screening tool we looked at in chapter 2. In order to assess your actual health risk, your RD may also want to look at other factors. For example, if your doctor is concerned that you might have a heart attack, your registered dietitian will want to know several things in addition to your BMI:

1. Do you have a family history of heart disease?

2. Do you smoke cigarettes?

3. How much physical activity do you get every day?

4. How much fat, saturated fat, fiber, and sodium do you consume?

5. What medications are you currently taking?

Together with your physician, a registered dietitian may request additional tests and lab work. All of these hassles can have a nice payoff if you hang in there. When I was obese, I didn't have the best opinion about RDs. I assumed their advice for me would be to "eat nothing but vegetables and learn to like it." After meeting several registered dietitians in the last few years, I am pleased to report they don't travel to work on brooms.

A good registered dietitian will actually want to know the foods you enjoy. RDs can work with you to keep as many of these items in your diet as possible and may have some creative ideas on how your favorite dishes can fit with a daily calorie target. Beyond your plate, RDs can also give you emotional support when the journey starts to feel never ending. There aren't many weight-loss hurdles these experts can't help you jump. They've heard it all! If a consultation with a registered dietitian is covered by your insurance (or can fit within your budget), take advantage of this resource.

Food should always be more than just calories and fat. You may know that in your head, but do you eat that way? When I weighed three hundred pounds, I didn't think about fiber, protein, vitamins, and minerals. I ate whatever could give me a quick hit of sugar and fat. I knew I was consuming too many calories, but I didn't want to face the actual numbers of my nutrition beyond that. My go-to excuses were:

1. It takes too long to read labels and think about what I've eaten today.

2. This whole vitamin alphabet/number thing is too confusing. A, B, C, D, Omega 3, 6, 9…whatever.

3. I don't need to pay attention. I'll just pop one of my kid's vitamins and that will cover me.

I was morbidly obese, and yet my body wasn't getting all of the nutrition it needed. A registered dietitian can monitor your diet during a weight-loss plan and keep an eye on important things such as vitamins, minerals, fiber, protein, and so on. Your goal is to drop the pounds as quickly as possible, but the organs in your body just want to keep you alive and moving. They must be fed.

My doctor has some scary stories of women bringing in bags of their own hair. These patients didn't realize that extreme dieting was robbing their bodies of nutrition. And if your body must choose between feeding your heart or feeding your hair, it's no contest. The goal is to find a weight-loss plan that can feed both. In my opinion there is nothing that can kill the joy of having a smaller waistline than trying to hide your new bald spots!

TOUGH LUCK ON THE EXAMINATION TABLE

After singing the praises of good physicians and registered dieticians, it is time for a quick reality check. Not all medical professionals will be a source of support during your weight loss. The knowledge of how to heal isn't always the same thing as the ability to heal. Here is what a good "bedside manner" should look like:

1. Your doctor should know when it is appropriate to talk about weight loss and when it's time to be quiet and take care of your immediate need.

You don't need a lecture about calories and exercise when you are bleeding with a gunshot wound. Hopefully this is an exaggeration, but I've heard some stories that are almost as bad.

Ann was a lady who struggled with overeating after the birth of her first child. She had been diagnosed with asthma, and the extra weight seemed to make her asthma symptoms worse. One night Ann's husband drove her to the emergency room of their local hospital because she was struggling to breathe. Ann was forced to listen to a speech from the emergency room physician about obesity and how it complicated the treatment of her asthma. A nurse later told Ann that her skin looked "a little blue" by the time the physician stopped talking and took the steps required to relieve her breathing.

2. Your doctor should have reasonable weight-loss expectations.

Drastic steps such as surgery should only be considered when all other methods have been tried and tried often. Here is another true story from the dieting trenches.

Mike and his doctor weren't seeing eye-to-eye on the best plan for Mike's weight loss. His physician believed that Mike's dieting history and body mass index made him a perfect candidate for the lap band procedure. This is a treatment for obesity where an inflatable silicone device is placed around the top portion of the stomach. Mike wanted to try one more weight-loss program. During the next thirty days Mike worked hard and lost thirteen pounds. He expected a round of applause from his doctor. It never came. Instead, Mike's physician continued to push the lap band procedure and offered to schedule Mike for the next lap band informational seminar. The doctor dismissed his patient's slow but healthy progress.

3. Your doctor should never use your size as an excuse to avoid routine tests or procedures.

You may need a blood pressure cuff with an upper-arm circumference greater than thirty-four centimeters, a longer tourniquet, a scale that can weigh patients who are more than three hundred fifty pounds, or an extra-large examination gown. These things should be provided without whining or grumbling from the staff. The goal is to find a clinic where you feel comfortable enough to come back.

Finally I need to leave the subject of health care with a disclaimer. There is no such thing as the perfect doctor. Everyone can have a bad day, including physicians and their staff. Schedules can be hectic and stress can be high. But if you consistently leave your doctor's office feeling "small" despite the number on the scale, it might be time to find another doctor. Weight loss isn't a quick and easy job. You will need a physician who builds you up for the tough work ahead. If losing weight is like a game of freeze tag, your doctor's office should feel like home base.

WHO CAN'T MOVE YOU?

As you are building a group of people to motivate and encourage you, it can be tempting to put people on this team who are going through same struggles that you are. There is nothing wrong with that in theory, but it can sometimes backfire when you put it into practice. The purpose of this support is to keep you going when you feel discouraged *and* cheer for you when you are successful. A fellow dieting veteran may be a great shoulder to cry on. He or she may know all about caving into cravings. But will this same person give you a pat on the back when you begin to reach your goals?

In my never-ending mission to "tell it like it is," I have some truths that aren't very pretty, but they need to be told. Not everyone is going to be a source of support. Not everyone is going to be happy about your weight loss. Not everyone is going to tell you how great you look or encourage you to keep up the good work. It won't take you long to recognize these individuals. You'll get comments and questions such as:

1. "Why are you trying to lose weight? Be happy with the way you are."

2. "You're doing this to get attention. You just want to look hot, sexy, whatever."

3. "Why are you so picky about the food you eat? Can't you just relax?"

As hard as it may be to believe, these comments have very little to do with you. Misery loves company, and it can be scary for some people to watch you make healthy choices when they are buried under their own lies and insecurities. You shouldn't take their words to heart, and you don't have to write them out of your life in order to lose weight.

Be sensitive around your family, friends, and coworkers. If your conversations about calories, exercise, and "pounds lost" are painful for some people to hear, don't talk about it when they are around. You can have a great cheerleading section without these individuals (even if the nonsupportive individual is your spouse). Your passionate speeches about calories, fat, and carbohydrates won't be half as persuasive as the changes they will see in your body. You will be a better advocate for healthy living if you quietly lead by example. And believe me, they will be watching you...closely! Your body is about to go through some dramatic improvements.

MIRROR, MIRROR ON THE WALL

We might be accused of being shallow, but go ahead and pull out your mirror. How has excess weight changed your physical appearance? How much different will you look when you reach a healthy weight? How will this "new look" be received? It's time to put our before and after pictures in focus and see them through the eyes of our spouses.

"Fernando" told us in 1985 that it is better to look good than to feel good. I wonder if Billy Crystal could have imagined how much more image obsessed the world would be more than twenty-five years later. It's almost impossible to avoid messages telling us that our pores should be smaller, our hair should be fuller, and our breath should smell sweeter.

As I stood in the checkout line at the grocery store recently, I was visually assaulted by the tabloid magazines lining the racks. Forget about getting my bread home without being smashed; these publications had a more important job for me to do. One magazine in particular needed its sharp readers to examine six half-naked rumps to determine which celebs had the best and worst beach bodies.

Quick side note: I'm pleased to report I cannot recognize Leann Rimes by simply looking at her from behind. I can also report that I had an overwhelming maternal impulse to feed the young lady a ham sandwich and a glass of milk. I had all of the ingredients in my grocery cart to make it happen. Sorry, I'm ready to focus now.

In order to explore the idea of a "beauty balance" within marriage, we need to take an honest look at our appearance. Thankfully most of us won't have our bodies judged on the cover of a magazine. Our examination will be a private one. I want you to look at your outer layer, how your weight affects the picture you present to the world, and how improvements to your appearance may impact your spouse. Let's begin with a close-up of how we look pre–weight loss.

Before picture: how unhealthy looks on the outside

When we think about the appearance of an obese person, we generally visualize rolls of fat, pockets of cellulite, and stretch marks. Excess weight can actually cause a long list of other external problems:

1. **Changes in hormones may lead to acanthosis nigricans.** These are the darkened, velvety areas that we sometimes see in the neck and body folds.

2. **Infected hair follicles can lead to folliculitis (also called barber's itch).** Small whiteheads form around one or more of the hair follicles on the skin. Obese people are at risk for folliculitis because their extra weight damages the hair follicle and creates an ideal environment for infections.

3. **Increased strain on the leg veins may cause fluid retention, leg swelling, the rupture of superficial capillaries, and varicose veins.**

4. **Retained moisture in body folds encourages the growth of bacteria and fungi.** This leads to some nasty skin rashes and a variety of infections, including tinea cruris (also known in a locker room near you as jock itch).

5. **Even our poor feet can't escape.** Obese individuals are more likely to develop corns and calluses due to their increased weight.

This is by no means a complete list of the external issues that go hand in hand with obesity. Our extra pounds can cause other problems, including gum disease, brittle fingernails, and even hair loss. From head to toe it's tough to "look mahvelous" with so many unsightly strikes against us.

I admit that I've been on speaking terms with more than a few of the external issues associated with obesity. I wasn't able to carry three hundred pounds without seeing some side effects. Thankfully jock itch wasn't one of them (dodged a bullet there). Finding creams, lotions, and potions to treat all of these "superficial" issues was exhausting. I eventually stopped trying. I used black, shapeless clothing and chunky shoes to hide my dermatological disaster zones. My decision was to forget about being attractive and settle for being invisible.

If it's been years since you've felt good about your size and appearance, your before picture may look a lot like mine did. The people who love you probably assume you have a very simple style or you don't spend time "fixing yourself up." Even someone as close as a spouse may not realize how frustrated you are with your physical appearance or understand that you haven't stopped wondering how you would look if you "just lost some weight."

After picture: how healthy looks on the outside

Weight loss is a powerful catalyst for change. Many of the appearance problems associated with obesity begin to fade. Good nutrition and exercise beats anything you can buy at a beauty counter. Someone who never seemed to care about fashion suddenly has a new haircut, some fancy duds, and bounce in his step. It can be a shock when a Plain Joe or Plain Jane comes out of the cocoon.

For some spouses this transformation is a pleasant surprise. Others see it as a threat to the "beauty balance" within the marriage. Has your husband or wife always enjoyed the unofficial title as the "more attractive" one? If you both carry extra pounds, are you currently a matched set physically? Your weight loss can dramatically shift this balance. Fear and insecurities (some as old as childhood) start to creep in and can lead to diet sabotage. Instead of providing the much-needed support you need to take the weight off, your spouse wants to keep the status quo.

To get a good understanding of "beauty balance" fears, we're going to take a quick trip back to junior high. Imagine for a moment that you are at your first dance. An Elvis love song begins to play (or maybe it was Percy Sledge, Foreigner, or the Backstreet Boys—pick your decade). After pacing, sweating, and checking your hair, you finally get the courage to ask someone to dance. There is a long, painful pause while you wait for a reply. It gives you too much time to think: "Does this person find me attractive? Is this person out of my league? What in the world was I thinking?"

Some of us haven't graduated from junior high and all of the social pressure that comes with it. The fear of being passed over, found lacking, or left in the dust can be just as strong as it was at the age of fourteen. These insecurities are most common among men and women who:

1. Were raised in a home where they were criticized for their physical appearance

2. Watched their parents go through a divorce

3. Have a painful breakup or divorce in their past

Your husband or wife may have "beauty balance" insecurities and not even realize the source of that fear. If you believe that you may have a diet-sabotaging spouse on your hands, it's important to realize that your goal to lose weight may bring these old fears into the light. Your resolution to look and feel healthier, however, is not the underlying cause of the fear. Odds are that your spouse's "beauty balance" issues go way back.

Like so many aspects of marriage, the key to receiving loving support from your spouse is to give loving support first. Stay with me through this next chapter. I have some tips on how you can build up a worried husband or wife. And here is a sneak peek: remaining obese in order to keep the peace isn't anywhere on the list!

Chapter Seven

LIVING WITH A DIET SABOTEUR

MEET PAIGE. SHE lost twenty-five pounds and just reached her first weight-loss goal. Paige's husband rewards her effort by buying her a box of chocolates.

Meet Mark. He wants to exercise more often and organizes a basketball game every Thursday night with the guys. Mark's wife resents watching the kids while he goes off to "play games." Meet Abby. She has been on a diet for two weeks, and the cravings are making her a little crabby. Abby's husband tells her to relax and have another slice of pizza. He likes his lady with a little "meat on her bones" anyway.

When I speak with men and women who struggle with weight loss, it isn't long before the spouse at home enters the conversation. A few people I meet are blessed with supportive husbands or wives, but most dieting veterans feel alone. Some even claim that their sweet spouses turn into sneaky diet saboteurs. What is really going on inside the head next to ours on the pillow? Do these men and women want to live with an unhealthy spouse? Is it simply a matter of ignorance or are darker forces at work?

BREAKING OLD HABITS

Because weight loss is a household activity, everyone under your roof has some learning to do about your new style of eating. The tempting treats your spouse flaunts in front of you may actually be the food lessons you've been unconsciously teaching for years.

Paige always loved receiving big boxes of chocolate in the past. Mark's wife had a tough day and wants to snuggle up with her husband and a bowl of popcorn just as they've always done for "must see" television nights. Abby's husband doesn't like watching his wife struggle. To ease her discomfort, he offers his wife a big "meat lovers" hug. A slice of deep dish always made her happy in the past.

The food classroom at your house is open every day. Through your eating decisions, your spouse learns where, when, and why you like to eat. Your honey also knows what foods you enjoy and how to use those foods to keep you happy. I taught my husband a few things when I was obese:

1. When Linda is tired or feeling stressed, offer to pick up dinner in the drive-through.

2. When Linda is happy, make an ice cream run and bring home enough for everyone. It's a party.

3. When Linda is upset, start preheating the oven. It's time for some chocolate chip cookie therapy.

The food education you've given your spouse can't be replaced by a healthier lesson plan overnight. If you've been heavy for years, one short declaration that "I want to lose weight" isn't going to cut it. Your husband or wife will need repeated, gentle reminders that your relationship with food has changed. It starts with your words, but it must be supported by your actions.

Saying "no, thank you" to tempting treats is a great way to begin the lesson. The real teaching moment, however, will come after you say those words. Be deliberate. Ignore the high-calorie food being offered to you and eat something healthier instead. Do this in front of your spouse. You may also want to mention how your planned treat fits within your daily calorie requirements. Make your point, but don't be obnoxious or nag your spouse about his or her choices. Lead by example and stay strong.

Will taking one bite of your spouse's "temptation food" ruin your diet? Probably not. The real damage comes from the message you are sending to your spouse. When you give in to unplanned snacks with an "oh well, a little taste won't hurt me," your husband or wife walks away believing that the new "food curriculum" isn't going to last. You may say you are on a weight-loss plan, but your actions are teaching the same old lesson. Always remember that your "student" is watching. Let your spouse know (through your words and your actions) that you are serious about making this change.

FIGHTING OLD FEARS

No matter how many anniversaries you've celebrated, one fact remains. You are married to a human being. Each one of us walks down the aisle with strengths and weaknesses. In a perfect world our spouses would welcome our healthy transformations and cheer every pound lost. It's the support that we need to beat the odds. And according to those odds, it's rough out there.

Most studies show that only 5–10 percent of dieters are able to lose weight and keep it off after one year. In the real world (where too many weight-loss plans fail) an unsupportive husband or wife can make this tough journey feel almost impossible. Let's do some investigative work and get to the bottom of this sabotage.

With so many health risks associated with obesity, why would your spouse want you to remain heavy? Did you marry a monster? Does the person who pledged to love you in sickness or in health want sickness for you? The reasons are more complicated than you might realize. I'm going to go out on a limb and guess you aren't married to a monster. You are simply witnessing the fear and insecurities your spouse brought to the marriage on the day you both uttered the words "I do."

After more than a year of anecdotal research (hundreds of stories gathered and way too much caffeine consumed), I found three common reasons for sabotaging spouses:

1. **Your weight loss could lead to a kitchen filled with nutritious food** (i.e., bland, boring, and bad tasting). Many spouses worry about having a health nut lose in the house. "Will my dieting spouse force everyone to live on celery sticks and wheat germ? Will this person want to throw away my snacks? Will I hear lectures and be made to feel guilty about the foods I like to eat?"

2. **Your weight loss could throw off the "beauty balance."** In many relationships the husband and wife keep a scorecard hidden in their heads. It might be petty, but it can also be powerful. When I weighed three hundred pounds and my husband weighed one hundred ninety, he was definitely the better-looking half of our marriage. Being the attractive spouse is a peaceful place to live. When we believe that our honey is "lucky" to have us, it calms our insecurities and fear of abandonment.

3. **Your weight loss could lead to extra attention from the opposite sex.** I wish I could report that this fear is completely unfounded, but I can't. Weight loss (especially when it is more than twenty or thirty pounds), can dramatically change someone's appearance. Added to this mix are often new and better fitting clothes, increased energy, and more confidence. It's a combination that can be appealing to the opposite sex.

If you suspect that fear (rather than ignorance) is behind your spouse's sabotaging ways, don't lose hope. There are some things you can do to relieve these fears and encourage your spouse to be more supportive during your weight loss. Let's see what we can learn from Mary and Craig.

WHO IS AFRAID OF A DIETING SPOUSE?

The story that I am about to tell you is true. I've changed the names to protect the innocent and avoid a lawsuit from the not so innocent. Your mission, if you should choose to accept it, is to diagnose the health of this marriage and discover what is really going on. OK, I've exhausted my supply of 1960s television show references. Find a comfy place on the therapist's couch, and we will get started.

Mary's not-so-merry Christmas

Mary was an overweight teenager who slowly became obese after getting married and having three children. Her husband, Craig, sometimes teased Mary about breaking their bathroom scale, but he really didn't mind her oversized curves. Craig loved his wife and enjoyed spending time with her.

Mary's opinion about her weight was less lighthearted. She minded her oversized curves a great deal. Mary struggled to find 3X clothes to fit her two-hundred-ninety-pound body and felt tired all the time. After some tests in the doctor's office she was told that she had impaired fasting blood glucose, a condition called pre-diabetes. Mary's doctor prescribed a plan that lowered her daily calories to two thousand and included some much needed cardiovascular exercise. Her doctor believed that weight loss would decrease Mary's risk of doing long-term damage to her heart and circulatory system.

It was a plan that worked. Between the months of February and December Mary lost eighty-seven pounds and finally fell below two hundred on her bathroom scale. Her goal was to simply "hang on" through the holiday season and ignore every smooth-talking gingerbread man she met. Mary might not lose weight during the last few weeks in December, but she didn't want to add pounds either. Every day was a struggle.

On the morning of December 25 Craig presented his wife with a large gift. After tearing through the wrapping paper, Mary pulled out a size 3X pair of sweatpants, several boxes of Twinkies, HoHos, and Ding Dongs, and a Christmas card from her husband. Inside the card Craig had written, "Please eat everything inside this box and stop losing weight. I want my wife back."

A case of cruelty or crazy fear?

The story of Mary and Craig is an extreme example of the diet sabotage happening every day within overweight marriages. It might even be the battle inside your home. I don't believe Craig presented that pitiful Christmas gift to his wife in the hope that she would do long-term damage to her heart or be diagnosed with type 2 diabetes. And if you are constantly "calorie tempted" by your spouse, your early demise is probably not the goal of your sabotaging sweetie either. Fear is a crazy, illogical beast. It can cause loving spouses to act in very unlovable ways. Your mission is to recognize the fear within your spouse when you see it.

Non-dieting spouses are often afraid: a kitchen stripped of all fun foods, a change in the "beauty balance" within the marriage, and too much attention on the new "skinny" spouse from members of the opposite sex. We are going to shine a light on these fears one at a time.

The anxiety that your spouse has about your changing diet and appearance won't be laid to rest overnight. It can, however, be slowly replaced by an understanding that the changes you are making aren't the end of the world or even the end to your marriage. The road to a supportive spouse starts by watching for the "fear signs," quietly working your weight loss-plan, and swearing an oath against whining, nagging, and complaining.

Believe it or not, sabotaging spouses often don't care what we eat or don't eat. The fear creeps in when our food choices start to influence the family. Spouses ask themselves, "What is this new 'diet fad' going to cost me? Will I be pressured to try foods that taste like tree bark? Can we still eat out, attend parties, and get snacks at the movie theater?" The number one fear that non-dieting spouses bring to the table has very little to do with our plates and every-thing to do with their plates.

Your spouse's fear: I have a health nut loose in the house!

The underlying concern is that your weight loss could lead to a kitchen filled with nutritious (i.e., bad tasting) food and an end to many of the activities you currently enjoy as a couple. Think about how many of your social events are centered on food and drink. It can be hard for our spouses to imagine going out on a date, spending a day at the amusement park, or even enjoying a night of bowling while you count calories.

It is not a coincidence that the majority of diet saboteurs are themselves overweight or obese. Fat loves friends, and your weight-loss plan may be seen as a threat to that company. To neutralize this perceived threat to your spouse, your weight loss will need to be a solitary walk in the beginning.

YOUR FEAR-BUSTING PLAN: FIVE DOS AND DON'TS

1. **Don't** try to change your spouse's eating habits in any way. Do quietly stick to your plan with a calm "no, thank you" when diet-busting treats are offered by your spouse.

2. **Don't** constantly talk about how many calories you've eaten (or not eaten), how many miles you've walked, or how many pounds you've lost. It may feel like an interesting subject to you. Your spouse will quickly grow tired of the topic. **Don't** give lectures to your spouse about the evils of high-fat, high-sugar foods. **Do** casually offer to give your spouse a taste of your lighter-calorie options. You might also throw in a few comments about how good they taste. Lead by example and not by nagging.

3. **Don't** throw away your spouse's snacks. **Do** keep them segregated. This one can be rough especially if these treats are also your favorites. Give your spouse a designated cabinet or space for junk food that can't be seen when you walk through your kitchen. Also, don't share the same snack space with your husband or wife. Putting your spouse's bag of cheese puffs on the same shelf as your 100-calorie bag of popcorn is a binge waiting to happen.

4. **Don't** stop participating in social activities with your spouse. **Do** find restaurants that have lighter-calorie options. If you are going to a party or an event that is traditionally a dieting disaster zone, quietly pack your own snacks. Keep it casual, and avoid making long-winded speeches about how "bad" everyone else is eating.

5. **Don't** use your spouse as a source of support when the scale frustrates you. **Do** find friends, coworkers, and other family members (outside the home) to build you up. This is perhaps the most challenging step in your fear-busting plan. It is also the most important.

At the beginning of your weight-loss plan, a sabotaging spouse can be like shark looking for blood in the water. Your weight-loss frustrations can actually give your husband or wife hope that this "wacky diet thing" will soon come to an end. An encouraged spouse will throw tempting foods in your path at a fast and furious pace. It can be a tough place for any weight-loss plan to survive.

If step 5 seems harsh, keep in mind what it doesn't mean. You aren't cutting off all contact with your spouse. Your husband or wife will still be a source of support to you in a million other ways. Love your spouse, laugh with your spouse, and pray with your spouse. Select someone else to cheer your weight-loss successes and listen to your frustrations when the scale isn't moving.

DANCE WITH THE ONE THAT BRUNG YA

I've started thinking of these people as weight-loss time bombs. Thank God these bombs are relatively uncommon, but they leave such a wide path of destruction that their stories can reach legendary proportions. Most of us know someone who knows someone who dropped a weight-loss bomb. We've heard the gossip. Plump Patricia becomes Petite Patricia and leaves her husband of fifteen years for another man. Big Bob becomes Buff Bob and picks up a girlfriend on the side. When the pounds start to fall, so do their marriages.

The most frustrating thing about these time bombs is the damage they can do within other marriages. As observers on the outside we can't see the emotional issues that might be contributing to the infidelity. We mistakenly believe their troubles boil down to this formula: Happy marriage plus weight loss equals affairs, abandonment, and divorce. Rumors spread about "newly skinny" men and women looking for love in all the wrong places. And when you announce a new weight-loss plan, your spouse may believe that diet sabotage is the only humane way to save your marriage.

If your relationship is strong, your spouse's fears may not seem logical to you. I can hear a chorus of voices arguing "but my wife should trust me" or "my husband knows I would never leave him." That may be true. You must recognize, however, that weight loss is a visual journey. Not only will your body change, but the way the world reacts to your appearance will also change. There is a battle waging between what your spouse knows is true about your relationship and what your spouse is starting to see.

TAKING A SWING AT THE FEAR

Pitch #1: A skinny slider

When you have success on a weight-loss plan, your spouse has a front-row seat for the entire ball game. You may not even realize how different you look. I know from experience that it takes the brain time to process a new, smaller size. At my heaviest I had to turn sideways to fit through my shower door. I've just recently stopped doing this—two years after reaching my goal weight. Our brains cling to old habits, and so do our husbands and wives. My husband still gives me the larger chair when we walk into our favorite restaurant. The "thinner you" will require an adjustment period so your head can catch up with your body. The same is true for your spouse.

Pitch #2: The fashion fastball

It doesn't matter if you are a twenty-year-old woman or an eighty-year-old man; you have the ability to make quick and noticeable changes to your appearance. Clothes, shoes, haircuts, and even your attitude can dramatically change the way the world looks at you. Once you lose a significant amount of weight, getting dressed in the morning may actually require more time and thought. As I slowly lost 155 pounds, I watched my feet shrink from a size 10 to a size 8, and I realized that tightening my belt couldn't save my size 4X clothes. I needed to do some shopping or risk "looking like a fool with my pants on the ground." The idea of a new wardrobe stopped being a luxury and became a necessity.

How does this updated closet look from the perspective of your husband or wife? It can be a shock (and not just because of the money you've spent). The person your spouse married—the person who often avoids cameras and mirrors—is suddenly paying attention to how clothes fit. It can lead to anxiety if your appearance is dramatically improving. Your husband or wife may start to wonder if you've changed. "What happened to my spouse, the one who has worn the same oversized Alf sweatshirt since 1989? Is my spouse becoming another person?" These are scary questions for some husbands and wives to answer.

Pitch #3: The curveball from the outside

This tricky pitch causes the most fear because it is seen as a direct threat. Your husband or wife might be perfectly content with your smaller size. Your spouse may even be enjoying your new look and smarter fashion choices. All of that will change the minute members of the opposite sex start to notice your new appearance. Suddenly the world is intruding into your marriage. It may feel like harmless flirting to you, but it will feel like trespassing to your spouse.

I can't find a gentle way to put this. so I'm going to speak like the overprotective mother that I am. Don't be blind to the danger here. It is real. I was obese for twenty years and couldn't even recognize when other men were too friendly. I just walked away and thought, "Wow, he is a nice guy who really likes to give big hugs." Someone should have bought me an alarm clock, because I desperately needed to wake up. Harmless can turn into harmful while we are still rubbing the sleep out of our eyes.

You have the ability to relieve the fears of your spouse, but it requires open eyes and open communication. The first step is to recognize your vulnerability. If you've been overweight for years, maybe it has been a long time since anyone (including your spouse) really looked at you or paid you a compliment. The first time it happens, you may be in shock. The second time it happens, you can become addicted. All humans are vulnerable to flattery. For those of us finally experiencing how life feels at a healthy weight, attention from the opposite sex can be an intense need that rivals any cravings you might have had for chocolate cake.

To fight the cravings:

- **Guard your environment.** Don't make plans that require alone time with a member of the opposite sex. Maybe it means that your office door stays open during meetings or that your business lunches include so many coworkers that your table looks more like an elementary school cafeteria. Maybe it means that the friendships you've had for years are now friendships with fences. Tell your spouse all of the ways you are guarding your environment. It will relieve some fears and also make for funny stories at the dinner table. (It turns out that teenage boys make wonderful chaperones. They can spot a "player" from miles away.)

- **Praise your spouse.** It is a fear buster that can't be beat! If your husband or wife has been divorced (or is a child of divorce), you may need to dish out the compliments and respect even more often. Your spouse said the words "till death do us part" during your wedding ceremony. Through painful experiences, however, this person has translated that vow to mean, "till things get irreconcilable, we drift apart, and you leave." You may not be able to completely erase these fears of abandonment, but you can begin to teach your husband or wife what being steadfast is all about.

- **Understand that flattery from the opposite sex is like a pretty package with nothing inside.** It's hollow. On the other hand, the gift of your spouse may look a little worn on the outside. Maybe the color of the bow has faded and the paper is wrinkled. Don't be deceived by how it is wrapped or the fact that you've had this box for a long time. It is filled with your memories, the struggles you've overcome together, and the knowledge that this person will stick with you through thick and thin (pun intended). Flattery is cheap and will never feed your soul like keeping the vows you made with your spouse before the Lord.

The Whole Truth—So Help Me God

During the last few years I've had the opportunity to meet several people who have amazing weight-loss success stories. They often look nothing like the before pictures that they show me. The difference can be shocking! And whether these walking "after pictures" are twenty-five years old or seventy-five years old, they tell a common tale. Your spouse, boyfriend, or girlfriend will love the transformation they see on the outside but may worry if you've changed on the inside. Be especially sensitive to the feelings of those around you, and pay attention to your behavior. Even the strongest relationships will need some extra care from you.

House Call With Nick Yphantides, MD

Question: You almost always had a copilot with you during your weight-loss road trip—family and friends. Why was this important?

Dr. Yphantides: During the darkest days of my initial transition—that first week—my father was the right man at the right time. He put up with the short-tempered outbursts, the nasty frustration, and the negative and critical spirit that passed through my body during the early detoxification process. Dad was a constant source of support, motivation, and affirmation. He did so with a selfless attitude of love and compassion.

Question: Do you recommend having one "go to" person as an accountability partner?

Dr. Yphantides: I actually recommend having more than one and giving them access to the inner sanctum of your heart. Your accountability partners should feel comfortable asking you the tough questions:

1. Are you sticking to your diet?

2. What have you eaten today?

3. Have you been snacking on things you shouldn't have?

4. How much did you weigh at your last weigh-in?

5. Are you still resolved to see this thing through?

Whatever form it takes, we need accountability. I recommend that it start from the very first weigh-in. When I started on April Fools' Day, I had nothing to hide from my brother Phil. I took off my clothes and stood naked in front of him. That type of accountability could have been humiliating and embarrassing, but I saw it as liberating. I was finally free from the lies and misrepresentation of how much I ate. It was an empowering experience that changed my life.

Chapter Eight

WATCHING YOUR WALLET GET FATTER

O N YOUR MARK, get set...hang on a minute. You are ready for your weight loss to begin. So stop and ask yourself, "Is my house ready for the journey?"

MUST-HAVE LIST

If you've been on several weight-loss plans in the past, you know how important emotional and spiritual support should be. It is crucial. But as I look back on all of my failed diet plans, it was often the practical, on-the-ground tools that were missing. You may have some shopping to do before day one of your diet. Here are the five items to put on the top of your must-have list:

1. A scale (buy one or dust off the one that you have)

This device probably seems like an evil machine of torture if you've been on a lot of diets in the past. My house went for many years without one at all. When I weighed three hundred pounds, I even stopped going to the doctor so that I didn't have to get on a scale. You need to trust me with this important step, especially if you have a lot of pounds to lose. The scale may be your only form of positive feedback in the first weeks of your weight-loss plan. You will need that motivation.

It was almost two months before a very observant lady in my office noticed that I was smaller. I had lost only about fifteen pounds at that point. I wanted to cry with relief when someone finally saw what my scale had been telling me for eight weeks. I was slowly losing weight.

After a quick search for scales currently on the market, I was amazed at some of the options available. Some models will calculate the user's body fat percentage, body water percentage, user's weight of bone mineral in the body, and daily caloric intake. You might even get lucky and find a scale that will brush your teeth and make your morning coffee. These high-tech machines are great if you want more detailed information, but they are not necessary if you are on a tight budget. The twenty-dollar scale in my bathroom gets the job done just fine.

2. Measuring cups/food scale (and put them within easy reach)

Can we have a moment of complete honesty here? If you've struggled with your weight for a long time, you have a vision problem. I'm not talking about being farsighted or having astigmatism. Your vision of what one serving looks like is broken. It's OK. My idea of "what makes one portion" was overinflated for more than twenty years. This condition is reversible!

Although I take responsibility for my vision problems, the food service industry helped fog up my glasses. Restaurants quietly redefined the concept of a portion size in the 1980s and not so quietly bragged about its growing portion sizes in the 1990s. The result was that America's picture of what a serving should be grew with every new extra, super-sized, monster value meal that hit the market. And the damage didn't stop at the restaurant's door. We took their standard of an "average" portion size and brought it home to our kitchens.

Combine oversized portions with the mealtime mantra we were taught as children (that cleaning our dinner plate somehow helps starving children on the other side of the planet), and you have a recipe for obesity. I can't blame restaurants for my obesity. I was an adult and clearly saw how much food I was eating. With that being said, I can tell you that my graduation from Happy Meal to Value Meal changed my idea of how much food I should be eating at one sitting.

It is time to learn what a portion size really is. Read the boxes, cans, and bags in your kitchen. If a prepared serving of Hamburger Helper is one cup, grab your shiny, new measuring cup and put one portion on your plate. Hold it. Look at it. Study it from every angle. This is what a serving should be. For my bigger guys in the crowd, you may be able to eat two portions and have it fit within your daily calorie requirement. Most of us need to stick with the portion sizes on the label.

3. Snacks (banished ones out and approved ones in)

The good news is that we're not talking about scrubbing the sink or sweeping behind the refrigerator. It's time to grab your "go to" snack list. Remove any of the "too tempting" items from your house and begin to shop for the healthier alternatives that made your list. More details on smart shopping later in this chapter!

4. An insulated cooler (or go old school and grab your kid's lunch box)

Even without meeting you, I'm guessing that you have a busy schedule and can't be within twenty feet from your kitchen at every point during the day. You travel, and your food will need to travel too. Before day one of the Skinny Budget plan, you will need to purchase an insulated cooler or lunch box. If your meals contain dairy items, lean meats, or low-calorie drinks, buy the small ice packs that can keep your cold items cold for longer. They are relatively inexpensive and will give you a wider range of eating options.

5. Storage containers

Most of us have energy and a big helping of optimism before the start of a new weight-loss plan. This can lead to some well-meaning but unused purchases that could be collecting dust in your kitchen twelve months from now. Before you spend money on a vacuum food sealer, see if shopping in bulk is a plan that works for you and your family. I recommend starting with simple, inexpensive plastic containers with lids, freezer bags, and sandwich bags that zip. Storage options that can be washed and reused are ideal.

When you have two or three months of successful bulk shopping, you may be ready to invest in a sealer that allows you to "vacuum" package meats, vegetables, cheese, and more in serving sizes that fit the needs of your family. After some research (with no kickbacks, money under the table, or tropical vacations to pay for my specific recommendation), the Seal-A-Meal VS107 received the good reviews for a countertop sealer. It generally costs about fifty-five dollars. The Debbie Meyer/Reynolds Handi-Vac costs about fifteen dollars and had high marks for a handheld sealer. Be sure to factor in the cost of replacement bags before you make this purchase.

I know the five items on this list seem simple, but don't underestimate how important they can be. It all comes back to the fact that you probably have a busy life and a schedule that is hectic at times. Your weight-loss tools should always be within easy reach. Do some shopping before you begin the Skinny Budget Diet. We need to spend a little money in order to save a lot of money.

A SKINNY BUDGET AT THE TABLE

Elizabeth is complaining because she doesn't like the stew. John Boy is in the middle of a daydream and stares off into space. Mary Ellen and Erin argue about a boy at school. Jim Bob builds a tower on his plate made entirely of carrots and potatoes. Grandpa cracks a joke, and John and Olivia quietly watch the chaos between bites.

This nostalgic scene of family-style eating on Walton's mountain is fiction. But if you've ever tried "multigenerational" dining in your own home, you know the drama can be real. It gets messy sometimes, doesn't it? Dinners with my husband and two sons are a strange and wonderful mixture of storytelling, teaching, conflict negotiation, culinary critiques, and burping contests.

If everyone walks away from the table with some good nutrition on the inside and a smile on the outside, I give myself an A. We were all fed and lived to eat another day. I've had more than a few evenings when the diners stomp off hungry and in a huff. Do we get points for trying even if someone leaves the table crying? According to the research, yes, we do.

In numerous studies family dinners have been shown to give kids healthier eating habits plus a lower risk of developing an eating disorder or obesity in the future. I even saw one Harvard study that examined the link between family dining and language development. Researchers believed that children with "book-reading" parents would develop speaking and reading skills at a younger age. The actual results of the study surprised them.

"What we found was that our data on the quality of conversations in mealtimes was a much stronger predictor of how later development would go for children's language and literacy development," said Professor David Dickinson in an interview with National Public Radio.[1] Eating in a verbal environment where adults and children constantly communicate gave kids a significant advantage over the children who ate meals in front of a television.

So how are things at your house? Is your dining table covered in junk mail and old bills? Do you remember how to turn on your stove? Take a moment to answer the questions below and examine an average week within your home:

1. Did my family eat at least five meals together within a seven-day period?

2. Were the majority of my family's meals eaten at home?

3. Did I prepare the correct amount of food for the number of diners at the table? (This doesn't include

planned leftovers. It does include overeating. You must answer no to this question if you or anyone in your family ate more than needed simply so that food wouldn't go to waste. You must also answer no if one portion or more was thrown away.)

4. Did my family come to the table with televisions, cell phones, iPods, iPads, game systems, and laptops turned off?

5. Did my family talk while eating, and did every member of the family participate? (Babies are exempt unless you want to count nonverbal communication. Flying sweet potatoes can often send a clear message to the rest of the family.)

Scoring: If you answered yes to the five questions above, the Waltons would be proud of your commitment to family mealtime. You have it figured out and probably scored higher than my family. I often struggle with the third question and preparing the right amount of food. I have two teenage boys, and sometimes they eat like children and sometimes they eat like NFL players. It's like trying to hit a moving target!

If you had to answer no to one or more of the questions above, you have room for improvement, and I have some tips to help you get started. Perfection may not be possible, but you will be amazed how your family will thrive with a diet rich in healthier food, livelier conversation, and stronger emotional support. That is our goal.

Lowering your food budget and the number on the scale

I'm going to sit back on this one and let the statistics make my case. A Zagat survey reported by CNN found that the average cost to dine out in America's largest cities is $35.65/person.[2] And before you argue that your favorite café up the road has more reasonable prices, even a dinner as low as $5/person is still more money than what it would cost to prepare the same meal in your own kitchen.

You must also factor in these "priceless" facts when comparing restaurant food to mom and dad's cooking. Dining out is convenient—no sweat and no cleanup involved. Preparing a meal in your kitchen requires planning and effort. In exchange, your family will receive more freedom. You will have the ability to prepare the side dishes you really enjoy, control portion sizes, and stay at the table as long as you like.

Want to eat your pizza with a side of grapes and asparagus? Interesting. Want to split a hamburger with your two-year-old? No problem. Want to keep the dinner conversation going for the next hour? Talk to your heart's content. There is no rush because there is no waitress waiting to seat the next family. You are in control.

Limiting your wheel meals

This can be a tough step if you have kids. As our children and grandchildren get closer to the age of eighteen, family meals can be challenging to schedule. My last two years of high school were a whirlwind of sporting events, school plays, and part-time jobs. I have an eighteen-year-old son who is in the middle of that tornado right now. He catches many of his meals on the go. I think it is God's way of preparing me for the day when he leaves for college.

If you are the parent of a high school student, a hectic schedule is probably inevitable. If you are the parent of a younger child, a hectic schedule is your fault. Dance classes, traveling sports teams, and play dates are fine in small doses, but eating fast-food french fries in the back of a minivan is a poor replacement for home cooking. If you or your child breathes a sigh of relief when an event in your family schedule gets canceled, you have your answer.

It's time to preheat your oven and give your child something healthier than food from a window and conversations between traffic lights. It's time to say no to all of the busyness and yes to more quality time around your dinner table.

A SKINNY BUDGET IN BULK

I'm going to be presumptuous and positively pushy and make a weight-loss resolution for you. How is that for bossy? Your goal this year is to eat more at home, waste less money on food, and find a healthy waist along the way. It can be done. If you've spent thousands of dollars on diets in the past, this concept will be a relief to your wallet. Welcome to the year of "buying in bulk without eating in bulk."

During the first few months of the Goff weight-loss plan, my husband and I tossed some big food mistakes into the shopping cart. Our motives were pure. We knew we needed to lower our portion sizes, and the food industry was all too willing to help. One-hundred-calorie packs and individually wrapped servings did the heavy lifting for us. The portion control was built right in.

When I was tempted to go back for seconds, I had to get up, walk into the kitchen, and physically open another package. It required effort and a conscious decision to continue eating. That "think time" saved me from more than a few bad choices. I was eating less food and losing weight. And even with all the good news coming from my scale, the monthly message from my checking account wasn't as happy. Shouldn't less food equal less money? Not necessarily.

I was paying a high price for built-in portion control. As a shopper with two decades of experience and 20/20 vision, this is a shameful thing to admit, but I had no idea what a unit price was. I thought it was information used for inventory control, or maybe what the item costs in Canada? The only number I tracked was the big number on the price tag—the one my cashier would charge me to buy the food.

Don't feel ignorant if you've never noticed the unit pricing at your local supermarket. Some smaller, rural stores may not post this information, or perhaps it's tough to see the fine print. After the whole Canada thing, I'm in no position to mock you. Stick with me, and you will be an expert. We're going to take a crash course in unit pricing because it is a must for smart grocery shopping.

Instead of the old-school method of putting the price for food directly on the package, the vast majority of supermarkets now use a horizontal tag placed on the shelf under the item. The extra real estate gives grocery stores the room to provide the actual price as well as the unit price. This second number off to the side is often a smaller font size or printed with a lighter ink color. Bring a magnifying glass if necessary, but read the unit price. Here is what that number will teach you:

Unit pricing is the amount you are paying for each "unit" (ounce, pound, etc.) of the product you are buying. We've been shopping for meat this way for years. By giving you a standard unit, you can compare apples to apples or more accurately cereal to cereal and cookies to cookies. A $2.49 box of cornflakes may seem more budget friendly than a $3.29 box until you compare the unit prices. Odds are you will pay a higher price per ounce with the $2.49 box. Every bite of cornflakes could cost you more even though you bought the box with the cheaper price tag.

Without the magic of unit pricing, shoppers must be savvy enough to divide the price of each item by the number of ounces or pounds within the package. If you have the time and patience for that, I salute you. My shopping trips were generally too rushed (or too lazy) for that much math. I shopped quickly and at eye level, missing the "bulk bargains" closer to my feet.

To give you an example with real dollars, I did some research at my local grocery store. This is what I was able to find by looking at the unit prices of some common breakfast items.

Quaker's One-Minute Oats

- The 6.9-ounce package (at eye level) was $1.00 and contained about 5 servings.

- The 42-ounce package (on the bottom shelf) was
  $4.12 and contained about 30 servings.

The larger size costs $3.12 more, but is it worth the bigger price tag? Yes, it actually is. The unit price on the 6.9-ounce package was 14.5 cents/ounce while the 42-ounce package had a unit price of 9.8 cents/ounce. The bottom line is I can save almost 5 cents on every ounce my family eats if I purchase the larger package. With most of the examples I found, buying a bulk size was budget friendly. I almost walked away thinking that "go big" should be the rule for economical shopping. I didn't need to look at unit pricing. I'll just grab the largest package the store offers and know I am saving money...right? It sounded like a plan to me until some boxes of whole grain hoops threw me for a loop.

Cheerios

- The 18-ounce package (below eye level) was $3.58
  and contained about 18 adult servings.

- The 14-ounce package (on an endcap) was $2.50 and
  contained about 14 adult servings.

This is where things got interesting. The unit price for the 18-ounce package was 19.9 cents/ounce, while the unit price for the 14-ounce package was only 17.9 cents/ounce. Because my boys enjoy snacking on dry Cheerios with no sugar (I swear it's true), I bought two boxes. It added up to 28 ounces of cereal, and I paid a total of $5.00. I am now a believer in the power of unit pricing.

You can keep even more nickels and dimes in your pocket when you begin to compare name-brand products with their "generic" cousins, become a coupon clipper, or investigate the warehouse clubs such as Sam's Club or Costco. A basic household membership averages between forty and fifty dollars each year.

Whatever store you choose, the goal is to save as much money as possible when shopping the interior aisles. Not only are you being a good steward of your finances (noble in and of itself), but also you are going to need that extra money. Roll your shopping cart along the walls of the supermarket and take a look around. This outer circle is where the good stuff is found, and it isn't cheap.

Foods along the wall tend to be less "messed with" by human hands than the bags and boxes found in the center of the store. Supermarkets often place fruits, vegetables, meats, and dairy products in the outer circle. When we eat the right portion sizes, these items are generally healthier for us than the processed items in the aisles. Unfortunately these body-powering foods are rarely on sale, and going organic could cost you even more. I believe it is worth the investment.

If you want carrots from a local greenhouse that specializes in raising vegetables to the melodies of Debussy, no problem. You've shopped unit pricing in the center of the grocery store and have money in the budget for "classical carrots." Interested in baking a free-range/no-hormone chicken that received weekly pedicures on the farm? Weird, but OK. You've found the best unit price on bread, peanut butter, and bran flakes.

A Skinny Budget Shopping Cart

We have a Baseball Hall of Fame, a Rock and Roll Hall of Fame, and even a Superhero Hall of Fame. Maybe the time has come for a Parenting Hall of Fame. The walls could be lined with pictures and exhibits of our children learning to ride their bikes, saying their prayers, and driving the family car. These are the wonderful "parent" moments that remain as clear in our minds as any digital photo.

Scattered among these memorable pictures would be the occasional shot of little Junior learning to tie his shoe or balance on the big-boy potty without falling in. Good stuff. Each milestone gives us hope for the future and the assurance that our child won't be the only kid in second grade still wearing Pull-Ups.

When I walk through this Parenting Hall of Fame, I notice that one milestone is strangely absent. We are missing a big exhibit (somewhere between the Tooth Fairy wing and the Sweet 16 ballroom). Where is the photo of Junior on the day that he became a participating member of our global economy? Where is the candid shot of him with spare change in his pocket, a sweet tooth in his mouth, and a chocolate bar in his hand? Where is the picture of Junior's first solo trip into the grocery store?

It is a life skill that is just as important as writing your name or driving a car. Both of my boys survived their maiden shopping voyage without doing jail time, but only because their ignorance of the law was accepted as an excuse by the management. I take full responsibility for their rough start.

I remembered to tell my sons they must pay for the candy before eating the candy (a prudent grocery store tip for children). I also showed them how to read the price tag and count their change. Unfortunately I forgot to mention that they can't pick up the candy and "run it out to the car to show Mom" before it is paid for. I made this error of omission with both of my boys, making it more likely that you will see their photos in your local post office (rather than inside the Parenting Hall of Fame).

We all had to take that first nervous/excited solo walk to the register as a child. We wondered if the cashier would laugh at us or ask, "Does your mom know you are buying this?" And after years of making our small weekly contributions to the economy, we each developed an individual style of shopping.

When I weighed three hundred pounds, my family bought groceries as if we were wandering through a county fair. Decisions were made spontaneously, and everyone tossed items into the cart. Some of you may have a technique in which lists are made, prices are compared, and pennies are pinched. Or perhaps you shop as if you are going into battle. It's a popular attitude among men. The mission is to keep your head down, find your target, and get out alive.

No matter what your individual shopping style, it is going under the microscope over the next few pages. Your planning (or lack of planning) before you leave the house, your habits and routines in the store, and even the way you put away the groceries can directly impact your wallet and your weight. If your goal is to be a good steward of your finances and your body, your work begins before you ever start your car.

Gone are the days of eating whatever grabs your eye on the supermarket shelves. It's time for a purpose-driven shopping cart, and I'm not going to lie. This requires time and attention in the beginning. For my family of four I had to dedicate about an hour each month to "food detective work" before a single shopping cart could roll (just two fewer episodes of *House Hunters International* per month). You are worth this investment, and you will get faster with practice!

Know what you are going to eat

Using free online resources such as www.thedailyplate.com or www.sparkpeople.com, search for your favorite foods. These sites have thousands of options, including "homemade" dishes, packaged foods, and even restaurant items from national chains. When you are considering adding a food to your shopping list, ask yourself these questions:

1. **Is this dish a calorie bomb?** I did a pre-shopping search for my favorite baked macaroni and cheese recipe. There were six hundred calories in each serving, and it had to come off my list. I didn't want to "spend" that many calories on a side dish.

2. **If this calorie bomb stays on my shopping list, do I feel strong enough to eat only half of the recommended portion?** In the case of the macaroni and

cheese, that would be a ½ cup *(prepared)*. I'm not sure if anyone is that strong.

3. **Is there a lighter alternative?** After a quick search I found a Kraft version of my recipe that is 385 calories per serving. I could save even more calories with a baked spaghetti or rigatoni.

Be curious and pay attention to the ingredients you will need, the recommended portion sizes, and the calories in each serving. Remember that your total calories consumed at the end of the day should fall within your daily limits for a slow, healthy weight loss. Know this number and don't guess! My goal was to eat two thousand calories per day at the beginning of my weight loss.

When I got stubborn and made meal planning a priority, I noticed some interesting changes within our home:

1. **I eliminated the "what should we have for dinner?" dilemma.** I had a plan and didn't need to pick up fast food on the way home or have a pizza delivered. This equaled fewer unplanned calories in my stomach and fewer unplanned dollars flying out of my wallet.

2. **I became best friends with my Crock-Pot.** On the nights when our schedules were busy, this gadget was faster than any drive-through and had better tasting leftovers.

3. **I sent a clear message to my family that I was stubborn about losing the extra weight.** Even my eight-year-old appreciated that a plan was a plan. When I told my boys I had a chicken defrosted, they understood that the clock was ticking. (Maybe they've smelled too many "Birds Gone Bad" in my refrigerator.)

Know that sales happen

I am a believer that having a weekly menu (that fits your family calendar and calorie goals) is the foundation for healthy weight loss. Remember to keep it flexible. Sometimes grocery stores will have perishable items on sale because the foods are closing in on the "use by" date. This can be a great opportunity to get a bargain if you put these items on your menu within the next few days.

Know that stuff happens

Broken appliances, electrical outages, unexpected guests, illnesses, overtime at work...the list of "stuff" that can happen to your weekly menu is a long one. Don't let an abandoned meal plan get you down.

Think of your food and financial stewardship as a game of baseball. It's all about averages. Sometimes you will take your best swing in the batter's box and strike out. Stuff happens. But if you can stick to the menu and reach base five nights out of seven, you have a batting average above .700. That is an on-base percentage good enough to make the Parenting Hall of Fame.

THE SKINNY BUDGET SHOPS SOLO

I've always liked a good party. Just ask Mrs. Fox, my kindergarten teacher. She would argue that Linda also liked an OK party and was slow to leave a bad party. My 1970s Raggedy Ann and Andy grade card even had a social category called "works well with others." I got an A (in the form of a happy face) for all four quarters by sharing my graham crackers and not sharing the chicken pox.

There were other standards called "keeps desk neat" and "works quietly." Mrs. Fox refused to grade on a curve for these skills, and some of the faces on my grade card looked less than happy. It was foreshadowing for the upcoming parent/teacher conference. I guess most fathers don't want to be told that their five-year-old can turn a classroom into Studio 54.

I'm giving you this information so you can understand how sorry

I am about this antisocial part of the chapter. I am a fan of family bonding, events with friends, and good fellowship (the word for a shindig held in a church basement). Have Crock-Pot, will travel!

As a longtime party animal, there are very few things outside of the bathroom I recommend doing alone. Grocery shopping is now one of them. And if you have children, this rule goes double for you.

I remember being a supermarket kid who begged my mom for candy and snacks every week. I grew up to be a mom who took her own children to the store and had to negotiate their pleas for candy and snacks. Even if you have perfected the "no, you don't need that" response, little shoppers make it tough to focus on reading labels and unit prices. Sometimes the best decisions you make in a grocery store happen before you ever get there. Grab your car keys, your shopping list, and:

1. **Leave your children at home with a big hug.**
   Share babysitting with the parents of other young kids or go to the store when your spouse is at home to watch the nest. Don't torture yourself by attempting a healthier style of shopping with kids hanging off your legs, surfing under your cart, or running down the aisles. You will feel like a brain surgeon with a Jack Russell terrier as your OR nurse. Our goal is to minimize distractions. We can't blame children for acting like "kids in a candy store" when that is literally what they are.

2. **Leave the passionate "snackers" at home.** This may sound like common sense, but it was a mistake I made for more than ten years. Sometimes the voice of temptation can be a spouse, but it is often a child. During the eighteen years of grocery shopping with my mom, I never begged for anything green (except the green clovers inside a box of Lucky Charms). You

know that walking away from high-fat/high-sugar snacks can be tough in the best of situations. You don't need a high-carb cheerleader on the sidelines rooting for junk food.

- **Leave the crowds behind.** Avoid shopping on Saturdays when stores are busy (generally in the late morning and afternoons). Also avoid 3:00 p.m. to 6:00 p.m. during the week and peak times before a holiday. A crowded supermarket puts pressure on the shoppers to just keep moving. We are tempted to grab and go so that we don't block the aisle or stand in someone's way. Your new style of buying groceries requires you to do the opposite. Stand. Read. Think. Don't be rude, but never let another shopper's glare push you into making quick decisions.

The grocery store is now your weight-loss classroom. It is crucial to break the habit of throwing "whatever looks good" or "whatever I always buy" into the cart. We want to push a purpose-driven shopping cart. Examine everything, and ask yourself these questions:

- **How many calories are in this item, and what is the portion size?** Let's sit down at the breakfast table for a quick example. When you read a box of frosted blueberry Pop-Tarts, you'll notice that the product has two hundred calories per serving. Good to know, but you can't stop there. The box also says that a portion is just one Pop-Tart. not the two that come conveniently wrapped together. It gets tricky if you don't read carefully—another reason to shop alone or with another adult who shares your desire to lose weight on a skinny budget

141

- **Can this item fit within my daily calorie limit?**
  It's back to breakfast for an example. A chocolate
  Costco brand muffin is 690 calories and will give
  you three grams of dietary fiber (the stuff that helps
  you feel full). A whole-wheat English muffin topped
  with one tablespoon of chunky peanut butter and
  raisins has approximately 300 calories and eight
  grams of fiber. Both sound tasty, and the second
  option won't force you to eat a dry salad for lunch.
  Weigh your options carefully.

- **Will I lower my cost per serving by purchasing a
  larger size, using a coupon, switching brands, or
  shopping at more than one store?** The "detective
  work" required to answer these questions takes time,
  but the effort can add up to big bucks. Before your
  shopping day grab the grocery store circulars and
  ask yourself if the extra gas required to shop at several stores is worth the money. Driving twenty minutes out of your way to save eighteen cents on green
  beans may not make sense, but driving that far to
  save twenty-five dollars on pet food, paper products,
  and pain reliever might be worth the trip.

We've been on a solo-shopping trip down the aisles today.
Research also shows that going solo is smart. *MONEY* magazine
conducted research on how often cash registers get it wrong. The
industry argues that scanner error cuts both ways, but *MONEY*
sampled twenty-seven major supermarket chain stores in twenty-
three states and found that scanner errors hurt shoppers more. In
the stores where *MONEY* "went shopping," correspondents purchased ten randomly selected items. In 30 percent of the stores
they were overcharged on at least one item. Reporters found

undercharges in only 7 percent of stores, and 63 percent of stores were accurate on all charges.[3]

You don't want to treat your local grocer like a thief, but don't pay blindly either. Some of the scanner mistakes may be in your favor, but many won't be. The biggest offenders are sale items, produce, and foods that aren't prepackaged—basically the good stuff!

To finish strong at the register, turn off your cell phone, keep the conversation with the cashier friendly but short, and find a spot where you can clearly watch each product as it is scanned. I personally believe we should speak whenever an item rings up wrong (either too high or too low). Most stores will honor the lower priced mistake, and you can sleep with a clear conscience.

THE SKINNY BUDGET SUPERMARKET SURVIVAL GUIDE

I want to stop for a moment and share a fact that is both interesting and ironic. Most obese people hate grocery shopping. Those born with a naturally "good" metabolism might laugh at this idea, but you know I am right. When I had a heavy body and pushed a heavy shopping cart, a skinny person would have watched me in the supermarket and believed that I'd found my mother ship. Shouldn't a big girl like me feel right at home on aisle seven between the jars of brown gravy and grape jelly? Not really.

Most overweight people will admit (when forced) that they enjoy the endless options of carbohydrates found in the grocery store. I was no exception. But unlike a quick stop at a convenience store, buying everything on a long list at the supermarket felt like work.

The concrete floors hurt my knees and back after the first ten minutes of shopping. The crowds made me sweat, and the narrow aisles made me self-conscious about my size. After more than an hour on my feet, I still had to push a heavy cart out to my car, shove the food into the trunk without smashing the bread or scrambling the eggs, drive home, drag the bags into my house, make room in my refrigerator (by throwing away the foods that were furry or had become self-sufficient eco systems), and put away the new stuff. Nothing could suck the fun out of the foods I loved more than a long trip to the supermarket.

What I needed was a grocery store training camp. In order to achieve a lasting weight loss that "played nice" with my body and my wallet, I had to replace vending machines, drive-through lanes, and convenience stores with planned and thoughtful trips to the supermarket. I had to find a way to make this work. You do too.

If your last adventure at the grocery store left you hot, tired, and in need of an anger management classes, I have some ideas on how to turn an errand that feels like torture into something that is tolerable and ultimately doable. Grab your tennis shoes, and welcome to grocery store training camp.

PLAYING THE GROCERY GAME

1. Schedule shopping at a time during the day when you have the most energy.

With extra weight on my body and a nine-to-five desk job, pushing a cart down every aisle in the grocery store felt like cardiovascular exercise to me. That's what it was. Don't plan a long supermarket run at seven o'clock at night if you know that your body naturally wants to hibernate after dinner. Less energy equals less attention to important details such as calories per serving and unit prices.

2. Eat a pre-shopping snack thirty to forty-five minutes before you start pushing a grocery cart.

I know you've probably heard this tip before, so I am adding some "meat" to the rule. Eat at least 250 calories and select items with protein and/or dietary fiber: pinto beans, peanut butter, apples, bananas, lean meat, lentils, oatmeal, and the like. You need foods that will give you some steady shopping fuel and not a quick spike and drop in your blood sugar.

3. Take a pain reliever.

If standing on your feet hurts after a short period of time, don't try to tough it out at the grocery store. Discomfort equals "let's just buy whatever and get out of here." We need to break that pattern.

Your new style of detail-focused shopping will require an hour or more of standing and walking. Ask your doctor for a safe pain reliever option, and be careful with prescriptions if you are driving to the store. (When codeine is the reason that your classic Camaro jumps the curb and crashes into the cantaloupe, I don't want to be held responsible for the new "drive-through" at your supermarket.)

4. Wear gym clothes.

I cringe a little as I write this because I've watched the TV show *What Not to Wear.* The hosts, Clinton Kelly and Stacy London, may not agree that tennis shoes and exercise pants are appropriate for the supermarket. I wish I could tell you to wear a fitted jacket that nips in at the waist, an A-line skirt, and a cute kitten heel. Fashion must take a backseat to comfort in this situation—and all the men without an A-line skirt breathe a sigh of relief.

Dress light and wear layers. The temperature inside a grocery store can change aisle by aisle. I usually start my trip with a zip-up sweatshirt. It helps me stay warm in the dairy section, and I can quickly remove it when I get hot waiting endlessly in the checkout line. Nope, no anger management issues here.

5. Prep your kitchen before you shop.

Open your cabinets, refrigerator, and freezer. Take a look around and toss items that are expired or have turned toward the "dark side." My shopping list often gets longer at this point. That's OK. It eliminates the mad scramble to save a meal because the potatoes I assumed were still usable now look like giant prunes sitting in my pantry. A rescued dinner equals no frantic calls to order pizza.

WINNING THE GROCERY GAME

Let's start by defining what a victory in the grocery game looks like. Your goal is to read the calorie information for every edible item that goes into your shopping cart, understand the recommended serving size, and buy the option with the lowest unit price. You can score extra points by reducing the number of prepackaged items in your cart, avoiding snacks that aren't on your list, and shopping the "outer circle" of the grocery store where the fresh foods are found. Here are some ideas to put a victory within your reach:

1. **Start your shopping trip by finding the nonperishable items first.** This gives you some flexibility with the clock. You don't want to feel pressured to make quick choices because your chickens are sweating and the frozen foods on the bottom of your cart are melting.

2. **Take a break if you need one.** This is another good reason to put the nonperishable items in your cart first. You are not a wimp if you need to find a bench, drink some water, and breathe for a few minutes. Like so many things in your schedule, grocery shopping will become physically easier with every pound you lose.

3. **Chew sugar-free gum and have a light snack waiting for you in the car.** This was my one source of sanity as I stood in the checkout line with a wall of chocolate bars on both sides of my cart. I'm not going to lie. Running this gauntlet and making it out alive may be the toughest part of grocery shopping. We've worked hard. We are tired and start to believe that a "king size bar" for the ride home isn't such a bad idea. Maybe eat half and save the rest for later?

You need some good ammunition to fight this battle for control. Put in a fresh stick of gum as you make your way through the checkout, and stay focused on the snack waiting for you in the car. Have faith. Those king-size candy bars won't always be such a king-size temptation. You will get stronger with every trip through the gauntlet

THE SKINNY BUDGET KITCHEN

Panic makes an excellent motivation for house cleaning. There is nothing that can light a Lysol fire under my feet than inviting twenty people to dinner. I clean with a purpose: beat back the clutter, the dog fur, and the unidentifiable "piles" on the carpet. I clean with a deadline: finish before the doorbell rings in three hours. I clean with a goal: make the house sanitary enough that guests will eat without a fear of contracting salmonella.

I could give you a tour of my kitchen after one of these panic-induced cleaning sessions. My ego would love for you to believe that my house always smells like vanilla rather than bacon, microwave popcorn, or a wet dog. I've decided not to cheat. I want you to see what a hardworking and semi-organized kitchen looks like. It has come a long way since I weighed three hundred pounds, but it is far from perfect.

There are some less than crispy vegetables in my crisper (I couldn't figure out a way to use the celery fast enough). There are two opened packages of flour in the pantry (I think one of them has sprung a slow leak). There are several uncooked popcorn kernels rolling around under my refrigerator (I have no explanation for this one).

And even with all of this imperfection going on, my kitchen has become my friend since 2007. That was something I couldn't have imagined when I was morbidly obese. I believed the lie that dieting meant staying out of the kitchen and putting a magnet on my refrigerator with a catchy slogan such as "taste makes waist." Wasn't this room the root of my problems and the dumping ground for all of my junk food? It was, but it shouldn't have been.

My kitchen was what I had created it to be: unorganized, under-utilized, and unloved. I needed a healthy kitchen to help me reach a healthy weight. As we shop as good stewards of our bodies and our finances, the final stop is putting away the groceries. How hard can that be, right? We take the food out of the car and find a place in the kitchen to stash everything. It is easy, and yet so easy to get wrong.

THE KITCHEN AND OUR WASTE

I could preach to you about how to organize your kitchen, but I think you can learn more by seeing my goofs. Many were the result of not having a meal plan or even a shopping list before I walked out the door:

1. **I bought items I didn't need.** It wasn't a big problem with canned goods, but perishable foods weren't so forgiving. When we started watching our calories and portion sizes, my family threw away a lot of breads, vegetables, and dairy items because I had purchased more than we could eat. Lack of planning equals wasted money.

2. **I didn't buy the items I really needed.** I thought I had milk but didn't check the expiration date before driving to the store. I knew that I had English muffins, but didn't notice the green fur growing at the bottom. Lack of planning equals wasted time and gas to go back to the store.

3. **I didn't take the time to rotate my "products."** This practice is standard operating procedure for supermarkets. The items with a shorter life

expectancy are positioned within easy reach (for shoppers who are in a hurry), and the foods with a later expiration date are placed in the back (a treasure for shoppers like me who take the time to dig for the fresher stuff).

Our kitchens need to model grocery stores. In my house it means that a new box of cereal isn't opened before the half-eaten box is finished. If you have children, this might require hiding the unopened box of Cheerios until the older Os are consumed. Adults aren't the only ones who learn to dig for the fresh stuff! Lack of organization equals stale food and waste.

THE KITCHEN AND OUR WAISTS

When you decide to pilot your own plate and pay attention to the food you eat, you have a choice. Obesity is so common that the food industry now packages almost everything in single-serving portions. You can lose weight this way. The trade-off is that you will pay a higher unit price for "packaged" discipline.

If Oreo cookies will be your once-a-month treat, purchasing one portion at a time may be smart in order to avoid overeating. If almonds will be your once-a-day snack, buying in bulk is a must. Bring out the plastic baggies and say good-bye to vending machines. We are now in the packaging business.

1. **Bag snacks immediately into one-serving portions.** I understand that you've just spent an hour or more on your feet at the supermarket. But before you relax at home, the kitchen needs some love and attention. It is dangerous to leave food (especially snack foods) in their bulk, oversized packages. We lose our perspective of what an individual

serving size looks like. Put on some music, kick off your shoes, and pull a comfortable chair up to the kitchen table. We can't save this job for "later." The overeating risks are too high.

2. **Involve the whole family.** Remember the children in your house who couldn't join you for shopping? Now is the perfect time to call the kids! Grab the measuring cups, a pile of sandwich or snack bags that zip closed at the top, and create a snack assembly line (with clean hands). It will be one less job for you and an ideal way to teach your children or grandchildren about portion sizes and healthy eating. These are just some of the foods that we package into single serving bags for grab-and-go snacks: grapes, carrots, strawberries, nuts, cookies, cereal, and trail mix.

3. **Be meticulous.** Read the nutritional information and understand the calories and the serving sizes. Measure! With our almond example, twenty-two dry roasted nuts are 170 calories. I want you to be confident that the zipper bag of almonds you grabbed at 7:30 a.m. has the correct number of calories at 2:30 p.m. when you are ready for a snack.

WHEN IS SPENDING MONEY SMART?

As I started to lose weight, I expected my wallet to get fatter as I got thinner. Gone were the late-night pie runs and the expense of eating so many take-out dinners from restaurants. We cooked more meals at home, paid attention to the nutritional information, and watched our portion sizes. So did I find a lot more money in my checking account at the end of the month? Yes, but not as much as I expected.

When you stop eating on autopilot (and when potato chips stop being your vegetable of choice), an interesting thing will happen. You will start to taste your food and really *enjoy* it. You will lose your patience with foods that can't deliver both good nutrition and good taste. Your plate will have three or four colors instead of foods that are just white and tan. Isn't it interesting that the God who created rainbows made the colors of the rainbow so healthy for us to eat? I love it!

And before we move on, it is important for you to understand that the rainbow, while wonderful to eat, isn't always wonderful for your wallet. Good food costs more.

When you walk through the grocery store and select colorful, fresh foods, you will notice something that might come as a surprise. Depending on where you live and the season of the year, your grocery bill may be higher than it was before starting your weight loss. This was sometimes true for my family even though we were eating smaller portions and buying more items in bulk.

I believe the economic reason for this "backward" pricing is simply a matter of volume. Because so many families are living on high-calorie carbohydrates, companies can produce these food items in large quantities, sell them at low price, and still make a profit. They are in demand and seem to have an ever-increasing sales volume.

Fresh produce, lean meats, and whole grains are harder to sell to a population that craves fat and sugar. There are often fewer coupons available for these healthier items. When you start eating foods that are naturally colorful, you will become a minority in your own grocery store. Take a look in the carts around you in the checkout line, and see if it is true. You are paying a little bit more for your minority status, but you are worth this investment.

If sticker shock at the grocery store has you reeling, I have good news. Some (or maybe even all) of this extra expense may be "reimbursed" back to you because you are eating fewer restaurant meals. We saw a nice savings when we started planning and cooking our meals at home. I think the food service industry in my small town saw a drastic decline in sales when the Goff family started using its kitchen (my apologies to the chamber of commerce). Keep that savings in mind as you are scratching your head and paying more at the supermarket cash register.

LOSING YOUR WARDROBE MALFUNCTIONS

I honestly wasn't paying attention. At some point during the twenty years of my obesity, baggy sweatshirts and stretchy pants with elastic waistbands made their escape. They were initially designed to be worn during exercise. In the dark of night, these items of clothing snuck out of the gym and into our daily wardrobe. When did these sad sacks become the uniform for busy moms?

Don't get me wrong. When I weighed three hundred pounds, I was the queen of sweatpants. I think I still have my crown. But as you begin to lose weight, this fashion choice won't be your friend. It will actually hide all of your hard work. It's time to set aside part of your budget for clothing that fits. We're talking about something very powerful here that goes beyond vanity.

It is hard to put into words how amazing it feels to step into a dressing room and walk out wearing a smaller size. Don't think this is just a "woman" thing. It's not. You can lose twenty pounds, and no one will notice until you put that smaller body in clothing that actually fits. It is a powerful motivation for women *and* men, and it can give you the strength to keep going.

If you love to stretch a dollar until it begs for mercy, you'll think about the expense of new clothes. You might even want to wait until you've hit your weight goal to buy new clothes. I agree that you don't want to spend thousands of dollars on a size 16 if your goal is a size 8. However, sacrificing now to "look good" later is a mistake. It robs you of the encouragement (and yes, the compliments) you will get from family and friends. It also takes away the satisfaction of fitting into a size you haven't worn in years.

It's not necessary to spend a fortune on new clothes, but make a small investment in yourself. It will pay off and encourage you to keep the weight off. There are several economical options available. Shop the sales, check out the "gently used" clothing shops, or find good garage sales.

To help offset this expense, look for places to sell the clothes in your closet that are now too large for you to wear. You can put the money you make selling your old clothes toward buying newer items that fit and flatter your body. Don't keep those bigger sizes as a "just in case I get big again" plan and believe that it won't matter.

Think of your weight loss like a poker game. It doesn't get interesting until you are "all in." By getting rid of those bigger sizes, you are officially "all in." During my weight loss, I knew I could either (1) keep the weight off, or (2) go naked. My neighbors are very glad I chose option 1.

All those old, baggy sweatshirts and elastic waistbands are a physical representation of bad choices and too many years of lies. Get them out of your house and focus forward.

The Big Price Tag to Remember

Our doctors have been telling us for years that obesity is a risk factor for several conditions, including diabetes, heart disease, stroke and cancer. If you are currently overweight and still classified as "healthy," the price tags below might raise your eyebrows. If you suffer from a disease as a result of your weight, these numbers may not come as a big surprise at all. You already understand the real-world costs of obesity, and your expenses may be higher than the averages below.

1. If you become diabetic

According to the American Diabetes Association, "People with diagnosed diabetes, on average, have medical expenditures that are ~2.3 times higher than what expenditures would be in the absence

153

of diabetes."[4] Diabetics average more than $11,000 a year in medical expenses[5] or roughly $225,000 over the course of twenty years. It breaks out like this: medical expenditures attributed to diabetes are hospital inpatient care (50 percent of total cost), diabetes medication and supplies (12 percent), retail prescriptions to treat complications (11 percent), and physician office visits (9 percent).[6]

2. If you develop heart disease

A person with heart disease will have medical expenses, including diagnostic tests, surgery, hospital and doctor visits, physical therapy, and costly drugs. According to the *American Journal of Managed Care*, the total mean direct medical care costs for patients with established cardiovascular disease (CVD) were $18,953 per patient per year. "Cost estimates varied widely, however, depending on the presence or absence of other health conditions. . . . Patients who experienced a secondary CVD hospitalization incurred annual costs that were 4.5 times higher compared with those who avoided inpatient stays. . . . Costs for persons who were not hospitalized for CVD during follow-up were about 30% lower than the mean," suggesting that "successful prevention efforts could substantially reduce the economic burden of CVD."[7]

Costs were also substantially elevated for those with specific comorbid conditions, including diabetes, chronic kidney disease, and depression.[8]

3. If you have cancer

Several studies have compared the cost of health care for patients diagnosed with cancer to those without cancer. A study reported by the US Department of Health and Human Services found that the average health care cost for cancer patients was estimated at $32,629, compared with $3,218 for individuals living without cancer. The report states that "a study of female employees aged 50–64 diagnosed with breast cancer reported the average annual direct cost associated with breast cancer to be $13,925 compared to $2,951 for a random sample of female employees. An analysis...estimated the lifetime cost for long-term colorectal cancer survivors (at least 5 years) were $19,516 higher than costs for individuals without cancer."[9]

Even with health insurance you know that the out-of-pocket expenses for hospital visits, lab work, and prescriptions can drain your savings and make living within a budget hard to do. You are taking a big step toward reducing these expenses by reducing your size. For the skeptics in the crowd I openly admit that we are all going to die of something if God doesn't have other plans. Weight loss is not immortality in our current bodies. It could simply be the difference between enjoying an expensive fifty years of life or a joyful ninety years of life.

Not a money person? Even if it has been years since you balanced a checkbook, obesity will cost you. When I weighed three hundred pounds, the price I paid was high. I lost opportunities, and I lost memories with the people who love me. Our family vacations had to accommodate my large size (no airplanes, no roller coasters, and no swimsuits). Our family table had to accommodate to my need for high-calorie foods with too many drive-through bags to count. Even our furniture purchases had to accommodate my extra width. Chairs with wooden arms were off limits, and don't get me started on the damage that I could do to a mattress. It was all to accommodate my obesity.

Eventually my eating habits would have cost my family a wife and a mother. Did I want the next generation to only know their Grandma Linda through an old photo album? It was where I was headed, and it was a price tag that even a "budget challenged" person such as myself couldn't ignore. Think about the costs as you make your minute-by-minute food decisions. Dedicate every smart choice to someone who loves you.

The Whole Truth—So Help Me God

After the first seven to ten days of any new weight-loss plan your initial determination may start to weaken. It will feel as if the honeymoon is over. People may even ask you why you are so crabby...just as my husband did! This is when you need to trust me and stick with your plan. It may sound too good to be true, but your cravings for sugar and high-fat foods will diminish. Your brain and your stomach will eventually "play nice," but it takes time. I can now walk past a box of doughnuts with chocolate frosting and keep walking. I would still be three hundred pounds if this weren't true. Keep going!

House Call With Nick Yphantides, MD

Question: When you decided to make a change in your life, you didn't mess around. Where did the idea of a "radical sabbatical" come from?

Dr. Yphantides: I went through much soul-searching and introspection. Believe it or not, I even fasted and prayed. I eagerly sought the counsel of advisers, confidants, family members, and God Himself. I believe the solution came as an answer to a prayer when I thought of the novel concept of combining something that I would thoroughly enjoy with something that would be great for my health. *That's it—going around the country drinking protein shakes and watching baseball games.*

Question: Did the idea of a change of scenery give you hope?

Dr. Yphantides: A determination settled deep within me. In sports lingo I would put it on the line, let it all hang out, and swing for the fences. I would pursue better health, a lifelong travel dream, and a baseball fantasy during an entire major-league season.

I thought of something outside the box to break my

loathsome habit of overeating. Habits are hard to break. Lifelong habits are even harder to break. Lifelong habits that provide immense pleasure are often impossible to break. My overeating habit had grown to such a magnitude that I had to do something way beyond the ordinary because my health was in such a sorry condition. If I didn't make its restoration the focus of my very existence, I would cease to exist.

Question: What advice do you have for someone who wants to take a "radical sabbatical"?

Dr. Yphantides: I was tapped out financially when I arrived home after baseball season, but I was incredibly happy and liberated because I knew I would reach my weight-loss goal. I was able to start earning an income as a part-time physician, working enough hours to "put salad on the table." I had to put everything on the line—my health, my career, and my financial future—to lose weight, and that was why I was so determined to see it through.

I want my overweight and obese patients to experience that same feeling. For some that might mean using all their vacation time at once—two or four weeks—to jump-start a weight-loss adventure. Even if they can get away for only one week or a four-day weekend, these individuals need to make it happen. Make the sabbatical fun. Take a trip. Get out of town. Expand some horizons.

Chapter Nine

LOSING WEIGHT LIKE A GROWN-UP

SUGAR CAN MAKE us fat. I think sugarcoating the truth can also put on the extra pounds. It's one of the reasons I refused to sugarcoat my struggles with obesity when I began writing this book. Losing weight takes wisdom and patience. You deserve something better than pretty lies that will leave you with a thinner wallet rather than a thinner body.

When I was obese, I was a fan of weight-loss commercials. I just knew that one glorious day scientists would find a cure for obesity and be willing to sell it for "three easy payments of $29.99." I'd just made a New Year's resolution to lose one hundred fifty pounds, and curiosity would make me drop the TV remote to hear more. Could this be the miracle I was praying for? After wearing out the numbers on my credit card, I eventually got savvy at smelling the scams.

The moment anyone in a diet commercial used the words *fast, easy,* or *eat whatever you want,* I put the TV remote back in my hand and switched the channel. Maybe I could find an old episode of *The Andy Griffith Show.* Both are fiction, but at least Deputy Barney Fife never needed my credit card number to nip something "in the bud." When the sun sets in Mayberry, shysters were either chased over the county line or sharing a cell with Otis Campbell. The same isn't true for the diet shysters.

I didn't realize it at the time, but my ability to smell a scam was a baby step toward a smaller body. I'd fallen for so many contracts, automatic debits, and low monthly fees over the years. Call me slow (or more likely desperate), but after two decades I finally learned that many of the promises in these weight-loss commercials could have been lifted straight from the pages of George Orwell's *1984*. I heard what these companies were promising and eventually understood that the opposite was often the truth.

Quick side note: I have a friend with an impressive list of acting gigs. One job was for a weight-loss company. Her image was used as an "after picture" for a diet program that this company was selling. The good news? She was a perfect example of trim—very healthy looking. The bad news? She's never been overweight a day in her life and wasn't an actual customer of the product. If the model is wearing the same bathing suit in the before photo and the after photo, you should be skeptical. The shenanigans of Photoshop may be at work.

These are the lies that you won't find in the Skinny Budget Diet:

Lie #1: Take this pill, drink this shake, or sprinkle this powder on your food, and you will quickly lose weight.

Truth #1: Healthy weight loss is slow weight loss. You have a much greater chance of lasting success when you lose one to two pounds each week through exercise and eating the right amount of food for your height, age, gender, and activity level.

Beware of plans that promise quick results by drastically lowering your daily calories below one thousand. Also avoid programs that ask you to entirely eliminate one of the five food groups (fruits, vegetables, proteins, grain, and dairy). It is almost impossible to permanently live with food this way, and losing your hair while you lose weight won't give you the most attractive "after" picture.

Your choice this year: Do you want to yo-yo for the next twelve years (rapidly gaining and losing the same weight) or slowly lose the weight over the next twelve months and actually keep it off? Instant gratification isn't always gratifying.

Lie #2: On this plan, you will lose weight every week.

Truth #2: I know that you learned in first grade math that 2-1=1. It is a clean and simple equation on paper. In the world of weight loss the math isn't always this logical. The subtraction of calories may not lower the difference at the end of your scale—at least not on a consistent schedule. Sometimes 2-1=2 or even 3! This crazy math was hard for me to live with during my weight loss. I had "dry spells" when I ate fewer than two thousand calories every day, and the number on my scale wouldn't move for two weeks or more.

It is at times like this when so many of us quit. We think the plan isn't working because our weight loss isn't in step with the date on the calendar. Don't fall for the lie that you will lose weight every week like some sort of machine. Our bodies are complex, frustrating, and also pretty wonderful. You will be rewarded if you stick with a healthy diet through these frustrating "dry spells." I had amazing weeks when 2-1=0.

Your choice this year: Will your impatience for results cause you to drop your goal, or will you hang on to it with all ten fingers? I can tell you from experience that a successful weight-loss plan is a stubborn weight-loss plan.

Lie #3: If you buy this diet program, weight loss will be easy. You can eat whatever you want.

Truth #3: If losing weight could be called easy, more than 60 percent of Americans wouldn't be classified as overweight or obese. A good plan will require your time and attention. If you see a diet that promises long-term results without exercise or a healthier eating style, you are smelling a scam.

The same ol' same ol' isn't going to cut it in a world where we avoid sweat and seek foods that are sweet and oversized. How can these tired, broken decisions lead to anything but the same broken results? I like this quote from novelist Ellen Glasgow: "The only difference between a rut and a grave are the dimensions."[1]

Weight loss for me meant jumping out of my food rut and blazing a new path.

Your choice this year: Do you want to let facts or your fears rule the next twelve months? Weight-loss companies understand that we are afraid of new things. Many use this weakness against us. They promise results without hard work or any real commitment on our part. Recognize the lie and understand that seeing a change will require making a change both physically and spiritually.

It can be tough sometimes to find the right balance between a faith in God and a faith in science. I always thought that weight loss would fall directly under the science category. I just needed one smart doctor to have a breakthrough in the lab, and those size 6 jeans would be mine. And while waiting for the science, I put the Lord on a shelf. The idea of praying and asking for God's power and healing in my life never occurred to me. Pretty sad stuff from a woman who believes that Jesus was and is the great physician.

If you are reading this book with a dream of what your life could be like without obesity, hang on to that dream with every bit of your strength. It is worth fighting for. If, however, you have a dream that someday a magic pill or medical procedure will make your pounds effortlessly disappear, it's time to let that fantasy go. It is not the Lord's will for any of us to remain slaves to a food idol—suffering and waiting for the world to save us. While hoping for a "miracle of science" someday, you don't want to miss the gift of God's comfort and power today.

In the Mood to Eat

If the month December is considered a stressful time for humans, August must be the most stressful time of the year for the plants in my yard. The heat of summer is when I often commit unintentional homicide in the front of my house. I have a theory that my jaded, old perennials actually warn the young annuals to "enjoy the water while you can. Bad times are a comin', my friend."

In early May I gave these plants my full attention. I pledged that this would be the year where my landscaping would live through Labor Day. A few months later? We have temperatures near one hundred degrees in Missouri. I'm distracted with too many vacation plans and back-to-school lists to notice that my plants are in a life-and-death struggle right outside my door.

I swear that I'm not a botanical serial killer, but we can learn a few interesting things about the way our plants respond to an unhealthy environment. Gone is the razzle-dazzle. After too many days of direct sunlight without water, my plants couldn't care less about their "nursery promise" to create beautiful flowers. They will even start dropping leaves in order to protect their crucial stems and root system. The goal of these stressed-out plants is to use any remaining water and nutrients to survive. Everything goes toward staying alive.

I would like to believe that I am smarter than the average plant, but I didn't always act like it. My go-to response to stress wasn't to fight for health. It was to eat junk. For more than two decades I would follow up bad news by making bad food decisions.

Eating was my ultimate place to find short-term comfort. Looking back, it was the equivalent of putting a water-deprived plant in a tanning bed—not the healthiest idea. Instead of giving my body what it needed in times of stress (the proper amount of vitamins, minerals, fiber, protein, etc.), I heaped more problems on my body with every pound.

THE SOOTHING POWER OF FOOD

Experts call it "emotional eating." In everyday language it's when we bury our negative emotions (stress, anger, fear, boredom, sadness, loneliness) with a fork and spoon. I'm sure behavioral psychologists have a lot to say on this subject. But as a former three-hundred-pound woman I believe our reasons for emotional eating come down to three simple facts.

1. **Food tastes good.** We have to be honest about that. Food also triggers a neurological reaction in the brain that we translate as contentment. I just read a study in the *Archives of General Psychiatry* that people who habitually overeat have a brain response to food that is similar to those with other addictions such as alcohol or drugs.[2] It involves the areas of the brain used in decision making, control of behavior, and learning the relationship between stimuli and response.

2. **Food reminds us of better times.** I can't eat homemade stuffing without the memories of my mom sautéing an onion in butter on Thanksgiving morning. It was an aroma almost as wonderful as bacon. Taste is the big player in creating these memories, but sight, smell, and sound are also at work. When an activity engages so many of our senses at one time, it is a powerful thing.

3. **Food was often our first form of anxiety medication.** Children can learn this pattern of behavior in the crib. Junior is bored, fearful, tired, or lonely, and his parents aren't paying attention to him. His plan? Cry like the world is coming to an end. The parent's response? Pick Junior up, hold him, and give him food.

We feed our children when they are hungry. That is a good thing. But to be honest, sometimes we will feed our children just to get some peace. As a young mom I quickly discovered that I didn't have a lot of willpower at two o'clock in the morning. If my newborn had demanded a cheeseburger in order to go back to sleep, I probably would have fired up the grill. I'm also sure my sons ate at times when they weren't really hungry. That doesn't mean every "milk-craving baby" is destined for obesity, but it's important to understand our pattern of emotional eating has a history. It's as old as we are.

Your first step toward breaking this long cycle of "mood meals" is to recognize the pattern for what it is. It's time for a gut check. The next time you step into your kitchen, ask yourself these questions:

1. **Do I feel actual hunger pangs?** If you have been overweight or obese for a long time, you might not even remember what this feels like. As an experiment wait a little bit before your next meal and get reacquainted with this sensation. Let your stomach ring the dinner bell instead of giving that job to your brain or the clock on the wall. Would you pass Dr. Rita Hancock's Apple Test in chapter 3?

2. **Do I need something to drink?** Our body is telling us that it needs something. Could you be confusing thirst with hunger? Start with a big glass of water and see how you feel in twenty minutes.

3. **If I'm not hungry or thirsty, why am I standing in my kitchen or waiting in the drive-through lane?** We like to believe we've matured since our diaper days, but our reasons for "nonessential eating" are often the same as when we were in the crib. Ask yourself if you feel sad, bored, fearful, tired, or lonely. What do you really need?

4. **Am I looking for a distraction?** Financial problems, work, relationships, health issues can pile on the stress. We feel like a withering plant in the heat of the summer. It is a painful place to be, and sometimes we wonder if it will ever end. At times like this it's healthy to call a "time-out" and take a break from the stress we face. But does our "time-out" always

need to be centered around food? Could we find another distraction with just as much enjoyment but fewer calories?

5. **After I eat, can I say I enjoyed it?** When we are in emotional distress, we often rapidly eat whatever is convenient without receiving anything pleasurable from the experience. In fact, our emotions can become so tied to our eating habits that we automatically reach for food whenever we feel angry or stressed. Gone is the decision-making process. Our eating is on autopilot, and we are just along for the ride.

Whatever emotions are driving you into the drive-through lane, the end result is often the same. The emotions return, and now you have the additional guilt of overeating. This can lead to the unhealthy cycle we know so well: our emotions trigger us to overeat, we beat ourselves up about our size, we feel bad, and we overeat again. It was the dizzying pattern of my life for more than twenty years.

I can tell you with 100 percent certainty: it's not the way that the Lord wants you to live. Stress is unavoidable, but maybe it is during our times of greatest struggle that we need less junk and more nutrition. Maybe reaching and staying at a healthy weight will actually lower our stress. Maybe we need to shed a few things and learn some stress-survival tricks from the plants in our garden.

An Invitation to a Crash Diet

Every time an obese person squeezes into a dining room chair with arms, it is understood that the most painful weight-loss wake-up calls don't come from people or charts at the doctor's office. The objects around us can provide constant, uncomfortable reminders that our bodies are too large. I've had several of these wake-up calls in my life, but the top three would have to be:

1. **Spilling an entire table of Thanksgiving food.** I would normally list this under the "accidents happen" category and move on. Unfortunately I cleared every dish and platter using only the reaching power of my rear end as I brushed past the table.

2. **Realizing that the table I just cleared with my "bottom power" was the dessert table.** Oh, the irony!

3. **Pulling the invitation to my twenty-year class reunion out of the mailbox.**

I have a theory that thousands of fad diet plans start with a simple walk to the mailbox. Thin people open a fancy envelope and believe that they've been invited to a party. The obese open a fancy envelope and understand that they've been invited to a crash diet. It's time to get thin quick. Pictures will be taken. Comparisons will be made. Who cares if we haven't shared the same air with these people in decades? If we can lose the weight, our former prom dates and ex-sweethearts will see what they've been missing out on all these years.

For a few cowardly moments I thought about throwing the invitation to my class reunion in the trash. The idea of seeing my old cheerleading squad in a size 26 dress made my heart ache. I quickly calculated how many pounds I would need to lose to look like I did in high school. It was a staggering eleven pounds a week.

I believe the Lord gives each one of us gifts. Rapid weight loss isn't a talent I've been blessed to receive. My pre-wedding plan to quickly lose fifty pounds couldn't withstand all of the bridal shower cupcakes and bachelorette party chicken wings. My post-baby plan to quickly lose one hundred pounds died during a marathon round of midnight feedings (milk for the baby and cookies for me). My house was filled with diet pills, workout videos, and meal plans. All had failed.

I did something important on the day I received the invitation to my class reunion. I said good-bye to crash dieting. I swallowed my panic over the upcoming event and took an honest look at my obesity. Did my body deserve something better than another frantic attempt to lose weight for the "big" day? What was my ultimate goal? Could I have a healthy relationship with food that was Creator focused rather than calendar focused?

Three months after pulling the invitation out of my mailbox, I walked into my twentieth class reunion wearing expertly applied makeup, three-inch heels, and a size 26 dress. I didn't apologize once for my size. I caught up with old friends and had a wonderful time. Maybe my three-hundred-pound body was the topic of conversation after the party, but it didn't matter. I was done with dieting to impress other people.

If the only reason you purchased this book was to "get skinny" before an upcoming event, my best recommendation would be to ask the store for a refund. Crash dieting may momentarily lower your number on the scale. The trade-off? It teaches your brain unhealthy lessons about food and exercise and dramatically increases the likelihood that you will regain the weight. I don't want that for you. Think about these questions and be honest when you give yourself the answers. No one is here except you and me...and I won't tell.

1. When I crash diet, does food feel like the enemy?

Instead of enjoying your food and looking for the right balance of carbohydrates, healthy fat, protein, fiber, vitamins, minerals, and so on—it's all about your race against the calendar. When you ignore nutrition and lower your calories at all costs, it has a steep price tag. You're hungry. Your body isn't getting what it needs to thrive.

If food feels like the enemy, it's time to call a truce. A peaceful relationship with your plate means you eat vegetables, whole grains, fruits, protein, and dairy every day. A peaceful relationship also means that you can eat desserts and treats. Diet plans that ignore one or more of these food groups (or expect you to never eat processed sugar again) are a crash waiting to happen.

2. When I exercise, do I feel good about what I've accomplished?

Getting off the couch (especially if it has been a long time since you've been active) is challenging in the best of situations. To turn a one-time workout into an ongoing pattern of exercise, you'll need to give your body time, patience, and some good fuel. A good starting goal might be thirty to forty-five minutes of exercise four or five days a week.

If you increase your activity level and get your heart rate up, feel good about your progress. Maybe you can't run a mile yet or lift as much weight as the guy bench-pressing next to you. Your heart doesn't care. You made a decision to be active, and your body is getting stronger because of it. Don't let a weight-loss "deadline" leave you frustrated or feeling guilty that you didn't burn enough calories. The only calendar to focus on is the one that is adding years to your life.

3. Do I feel like the pounds are dropping too slowly?

This is perhaps the most damaging attitude that can come from crash dieting. I've seen too many people put their heart into losing weight and walk away disappointed because they lost "only" two pounds this week. Gone is the feeling of accomplishment that should come from moving in the right direction. It's all about being thinner for that one important day. During my weight loss, a two-pound drop was cause for a celebration. If your weight-loss deadline is stealing that joy, it is a bad idea.

4. What will I eat the day after?

After a crash diet has ended, it is human nature to celebrate a little bit and relax. The "big day" is over, the pictures are on Facebook, and the dress clothes are back in the closet. Do you plan to start "eating normal" again? And is your definition of normal broken? How many times do you want to gain and lose the same weight?

A vast majority of crash diets teach you nothing about how to eat in the real world. They prey on your insecurities and impatience. They give you short-term results rather than long-term health. Grab some string because you are a yo-yo dieter in the making.

5. Would I put someone I love on this plan?

This is the final question and perhaps the most enlightening. Fighting obesity is just that…a fight. Would you send someone you love into this battle with a weapon that is painful to carry and likely to backfire? Would you give the person you love a flawed plan that will provide a momentary victory but be followed by a lifetime of defeat? And if you wouldn't choose this for someone you love, why would you decide to fight obesity this way?

MAY CAUSE DRY MOUTH AND CONSTIPATION

When my husband and I see an advertisement for a new prescription drug on television, we play a little game that I'd like to recommend. You quickly call out three side effects and wait to see if they match the adverse effects rattled off at the end of the commercial. It is one point for every "complaint" you get correct. I've had a lot of luck lately with "dry mouth," "constipation," and "a sudden drop in blood pressure."

After a particularly long list of side effects I start to wonder why anyone would actually give money to a pharmacy just to be tortured. It's really a statement of how far people will go to find relief. They weigh their illness against the list of possible adverse reactions from a new medication and decide to take a chance. If I had severe pain or a condition that was taking away my quality of life, I'd take the gamble too. Desperate times call for desperate measures.

I'd like to give you a short quiz and see how many side effects you would be willing to withstand. You have an on-going health condition that has become life threatening. As you watch a male model on television romp on the beach with a couple of puppies, a soothing voice delivers the good news. There is a cure for what ails you. Unfortunately this miracle of science also comes with some bad news. "This drug may cause dehydration, gallstones, electrolyte imbalances (which in rare cases may be life threatening), malnutrition, headaches, irritability, fatigue, and dizziness."

Are you still with me? Still willing to try this prescription? OK, let's continue. "This drug may also cause menstrual irregularities, constipation, muscle loss, and hair loss." Whew, this must be some kind of medicine. What disease could be so bad that a person would be willing to suffer through this many side effects to find relief? Obesity.

These are just some of the adverse reactions that can result from a prolonged "rapid weight-loss" diet (an extreme reduction in calories that is sometimes combined with exercise). It is the ultimate example of desperate times calling for desperate measures. And as a former desperate person who needed to lose more than one hundred fifty pounds, I understand the hopelessness that drives obese people toward drastic solutions. I have a long list of "drastic" in my past—all without much success.

When we are sitting on our couches (sometimes decades into our obesity), it can be almost impossible to look at our overeating and its impact on our health with any degree of clarity. If losing thirty pounds in three months is good, we believe that losing thirty pounds in three weeks is even better. Sign me up for whatever will get me out of these size 24 jeans before the next class reunion. Does your weight-loss calendar look like the property of a sensible adult or a child who "wants what she wants and wants it now"? Grown-up expectations lead to lasting, grown-up weight loss.

FAT JOKES AND MEAN GIRL MOTIVATIONS

Please raise your right hand and take this oath with me: I will read the following information in a spirit of maturity. I will not repeat the jokes or use the material in order to get a laugh at someone else's expense. And with that small bit of housekeeping out of the way, let's get started.

My maiden name is Brown. There are thousands of people in the United States with the same last name. It seemed harmless when I was a little girl, and I didn't mind having a name that was also a color. Betty White had blazed a trail for all of us.

I was able to live peacefully with a pigmented last name until high school. Harmless turned into harmful the day that a young man yelled, "How now brown cow!" down a crowded hall between classes. It was the first time that anyone really paid attention to my slightly oversized shape, and the clever phrase caught on.

The "Brown Cow" laughed along with everyone else in the eleventh grade, and the rhyming line ran its natural course through the high school. A few weeks later some other poor person (maybe with a bad haircut or smelly feet) became the new punch line to everyone's jokes.

The laughs got a little louder in college. A group of guys in my marching band placed my name on an interesting list. In the classic David Letterman style I was number five in a ranking of "the top ten people we would least like to see in a bathing suit." This list was distributed one Saturday afternoon during the third quarter of a football game. Band students aren't known for having rock-hard bodies, so a number five ranking in an organization with hundreds of members was a dubious honor. The "anti-swimsuit model" laughed along with everyone else and kept marching.

Men and their fat jokes

I've heard some interesting fat jokes over the last twenty years. My favorite might be that when I go to the beach, the whales serenade me with "We Are Family." I had to give this guy extra points for working Sister Sledge into the punch line. There are exceptions, but fat jokes are generally created, collected, and circulated by men.

I want to stop and say for the record that this isn't a "poor me" message. No matter what a person's size or shape, we've all felt the stings of group laughter. Maybe you have a big nose, bowed legs, or a bald spot. Among men the ability to take a joke is essential. It means that you are a part of the pack. And as a pack member you are expected to throw a few rude comments back in response.

Ladies, it is true that some fat jokes come from the mouths of truly mean men, but most leave the lips of guys who are simply looking for laughs. These stand-up comedians believe that:

1. **A joke about your size is no big deal.** After all, these guys don't care if their friends make fun of how they look every now and then. (When the teasing goes too far, threats of physical retaliation will generally send the required message and clear the air.)

2. **Humor is status.** A fat joke might upset you for a few minutes, but a long, loud laugh from the other guys make it worth the risk. These men underestimate the months (and even the years) that these comments can roll around inside a woman's brain.

3. **If the jokes bother you that much, stop being so sensitive or lose the weight.** Most men are action oriented. It is difficult for guys to understand why a woman would feel insecure about her extra pounds but not work to fix the problem. (It is a simple logic that is hard to argue against.)

It's not that women can't see obesity in other people. We can. We simply don't think that it is funny. Some of us kick into maternal mode and start recommending diet plans and exercise routines (torture for obese people who don't want to hear it). Other ladies have no patience for maternal. When they see an overweight person, they go mean.

Women and their fat contempt

CBS debuted *Mike & Molly* in 2010. This is a sitcom about an overweight couple who met at an Overeater's Anonymous meeting and start dating. The characters of Mike and Molly are romantic and aren't shy about hugging and kissing. Their premarital activities on camera are the same as other "heavy petting" sitcom couples on television, but it's the first time that a major network has shown an obese man and woman being intimate every week.

Blame it on my own years of obesity, but I wasn't shocked to hear about a post written by *Marie Claire* magazine blogger Maura Kelly. It was titled "Should Fatties Get a Room? (Even on TV)," and she asks her readers if people are uncomfortable watching an obese couple make out on television.[3]

"Yes, I think I'd be grossed out if I had to watch two characters with rolls and rolls of fat kissing each other...because I'd be grossed out if I had to watch them doing anything," she writes in her post. "To be brutally honest, even in real life, I find it aesthetically displeasing to watch a very, very fat person simply walk across a room—just like I'd find it distressing if I saw a very drunk person stumbling across a bar or a heroin addict slumping in a chair."[4]

At the end of her post, Kelly asks, "Fat people making out on TV—are you cool with it? Do you think I'm being an insensitive jerk?" She quickly got an answer. Within three days of her post, Kelly received nearly one thousand outraged comments from readers. The reaction to her post was so strong that Kelly issued a response and apologized for her insensitivity.

"A few commenters and one of my friends mentioned that my extreme reaction might have grown out of my own body issues, my history as an anorexic, and my life-long obsession with being thin...I think that's an accurate insight," Kelly explained.[5]

Like with so many nasty thoughts and feelings, we shouldn't be surprised to discover that fear was lingering right below the surface. "Mean women" such as Kelly are often insecure women. They obsess about their own physical appearances and are quick to put themselves in another person's oversized body. "What if I was obese? Would men still find me attractive? How would being 'fat' change my life?"

The answers to those questions can be scary. The "mean" learn to cover their fat fears with contempt for the obese. It is simply a shield. In fact, I often meet overweight women who have more self-confidence and peace than their "mean but lean" counterparts. These large ladies might understand that they have some weight to lose, but also understand that they have value in the eyes of the Lord.

Should jokesters and mean girls drive you?

During the twenty years of my obesity I started at least a handful of weight-loss plans because of an encounter with a fat joke or a "mean girl." Pain can be a powerful motivator. It is also a passing motivator. Healthy journeys can't be sustained by unhealthy abuse. Who wants to take a long trip with a driver who beats you down with crude jokes or cruel comments? Eventually even the most peaceful among us will leave these hurtful men and women in a ditch by the side of the road and turn the car around. As you start the Skinny Budget Diet, look for weight-loss motivations that bring you joy.

WOMEN CHASING PRETTY

This section of the chapter isn't going as I planned. For months I've been looking at the media and the body image messages that invade our homes through television, magazines, the Internet, and video games. It's a *Toddlers & Tiaras'* world, and we are "crowning" the wrong values. My goal this week was to dive into these questions: What is the media teaching our children and grandchildren? Is the next generation of women learning to value "skinny and beautiful" above all else? Can caring adults give our kids another viewpoint?

There is an old cliché that when you point your finger at someone else, most of the fingers on your hand are pointing back at you. I'd like to kick the person who first discovered that little piece of homespun wisdom. It's a humbling truth to accept. My indictment of the media and its evil messages became something completely different. I noticed how many fingers were pointing back at me.

My husband and I have the pleasure (and the occasional pain) of teaching a first grade Sunday school class in our church. In my defense I must go on the record as saying they are an attractive bunch of children, and we see these kids at their best. They come through our classroom door with clean faces, combed hair, and some stylish choices. The children may not leave looking as shiny (unless our craft project uses glitter), but they look great when we first greet them. That is my problem.

When a young boy walks into our class on a Sunday morning, we put a sticker on the attendance chart and start a conversation about his week. I might ask about school, his sports teams, or if he finally lost that loose tooth. The "greeting procedure" starts the same when a young girl walks into the room. We put a sticker on the attendance chart and start a conversation. That is where the similarities end.

Over and over again I noticed that my go-to topics with a little girl were:

1. Her pretty hair (Wow, I love the bows.)

2. Her pretty dress (The fabric really sparkles. Do you think that dress comes in my size?)

3. Her pretty shoes (A great color. Do you think those shoes come in my size?)

We might get around to discussing school, hobbies, and exciting visits from the Tooth Fairy, but first things first. I must notice the outside. I must make her feel welcome by giving her compliments about her physical appearance. I must reassure her that she passed the inspection of the adults in the room.

Every word we say in front of a child is important, but the first words we speak are the most powerful. They communicate our priorities. They give a clear indication of our preferences, expectations, and what we value. When used properly, these words will recognize the traits that make the child standing in front of us unique—his or her creativity, intellect, talent, and character. I have been wasting that precious opportunity with these young girls and leaving some potentially damaging messages in its place.

When I greet a young lady with a "you look so pretty today" comment, I'm actually giving a nod to my own history of body image issues. I want this child to feel good about her appearance because I didn't always feel that way. I want her to have self-confidence because mine was sometimes lacking. I want her to like what she sees in the mirror because I often didn't when I was growing up. I have the best of intentions...so what's so wrong with starting a conversation with a girl this way? It turns out that this road of good intentions has some big potholes.

1. Wrong priorities

With our "pretty" compliments, we communicate a not-so-subtle message to the girl in front of us (and the other young ladies within earshot) that this is what makes a female valuable. We also send a loud message to the boys in the room that a woman's personality, abilities, and character are secondary. It's all about the external picture that she presents to the world. It's all about meeting whatever today's standard of thin and beautiful might be. Unfortunately it can also be all about pain if and when the compliments stop coming. Will she have the confidence to see that God wraps our gifts and talents in boxes—boxes that come in all shapes and sizes, boxes that get wrinkled when they get wisdom, boxes that are unique and beautiful in God's eyes?

2. Wasted potential

This one comes with a story that I'm not proud to tell. At the age of eighteen I was a high school writer who also liked public speaking. Broadcast journalism seemed like an ideal career choice for me. I received a scholarship and was accepted into the journalism school after my sophomore year at the University of Missouri. It was an outstanding program. I learned how to write an inverted pyramid, how to protect my sources, and even a few things about journalistic ethics (I'll let you decide if this is an oxymoron).

During my final year of college the day came for "on-air" evaluations. My professor watched each one of his students in front of the camera and gave us an individualized critique. In a room filled with other hopeful journalists, I was told that my look "wasn't professional enough" for television. Because of my physical appearance and the extra fifty pounds I was carrying, my professor believed it would be difficult for me to find a job in front of the camera. It's a tough thing to hear that you have a face for radio when you are a twenty-two-year-old woman.

I dropped out of the journalism program just six hours short of graduation. And while this may sound like a "shame on the professor" story, it is actually a "shame on me" story. I believed a lie. I believed that the gifts and talents I had on the inside meant nothing without a pretty package on the outside. I believed that potential employers would take one look at an overweight, female reporter and say "no, thanks."

3. Worldly perfection

When we teach the next generation of women to crave pretty compliments and chase our culture's idea of beauty, we are sending them on a race that doesn't have a finish line. Few of us can actually achieve the world's idea of external "beauty," and none of us can keep it for long. I started too many weight-loss plans trying to be the fickle world's definition of "pretty." It was exhausting. As adult women we need to stop running this race, stop blaming the media, and stop passing our insecurities on to the next generation.

I recently took my first step. I had a conversation with every young girl in my Sunday school class and didn't use the word "pretty" once. We read Max Lucado's book *If Only I Had a Green Nose* and talked about how we are each created as a one-of-a-kind.[6] The Lord made something complex and wonderful when He took a rib from Adam. It is an important message for six-year-old girls to hear—and a healthy reminder for the forty-something in the room too.

Chapter Ten

TAKING YOUR PLAN ON THE ROAD

I F LOSING WEIGHT feels like a war, dining out without consuming thousands of extra calories is like storming the beaches of Normandy. It is dangerous. There can be traps. It will require knowledge and a stubborn spirit to survive.

When I started my weight loss, I decided that restaurants would be off-limits. I didn't want to ruin days of hard work with an hour of high-calorie dishes that I would regret eating later. I knew that losing one hundred fifty pounds would be hard enough in my own house. But try to make healthier eating decisions in the face of endless breadsticks, deep-dish pizzas and chocolate lava cakes? It couldn't be done. Restaurants of any kind were forbidden. And I am proud to report that I held firm to my resolution...for about two weeks.

I have a husband, two children, wonderful friends, and a job that requires me to travel several times a week. My oath of never eating in restaurants was well meaning but naïve. There may be a few of you reading this chapter who can't remember the last time you ate a meal anywhere but in the comfort of your own home. Congratulations. You are as unique and rare as a purple cat. For most of us restaurant food is a part of life. It is a place for celebrations, meeting friends, getting some business done, and grabbing a quick bite on the run. In order to develop a better relationship with food, you must be able to occasionally walk into a restaurant and make it out alive.

My fear of dining out had to be replaced with a healthy attitude of caution. Restaurant food could be a part of my weight-loss plan, but it had to be on my terms. I began thinking of the menu as a starting point. It was a tool I had to customize. The day I had the courage to ask for soup instead of french fries (a switch that wasn't on the menu), I expected my waitress to stomp off in a huff. It never happened. She didn't even blink when I hollowed-out my hamburger bun and left one-third of its calories on my plate.

By the time I got my bill, the waitress had probably forgotten all about my "strange" behavior at the table. I was polite about my requests and left a decent tip. That is generally all it takes to get a server on your side for future visits. Don't be afraid or embarrassed to "go rogue" from the choices on the menu. Your waiter or waitress might have their own healthy suggestions if you ask for them.

Did you ever see the 1989 movie *When Harry Met Sally*? At 300 pounds I thought Sally's style of ordering food was ridiculous. At 145 pounds I've decided that her method of customizing a plate was genius.

> Sally Albright: But I'd like the pie heated, and I don't want the ice cream on top. I want it on the side, and I'd like strawberry instead of vanilla, if you have it. If not, then no ice cream just whipped cream, but only if it's real. If it's out of a can, then nothing.
>
> Waitress: Not even the pie?
>
> Sally Albright: No, just the pie, but then not heated.[1]

What can we learn from this…other than the many ways you can order a pie? Don't let the restaurant call the shots. Your weight-loss battle plan must travel with you into the restaurant. There may be a section on the menu with "healthy" suggestions, but don't count on it. You must enter this war zone with some thorough reconnaissance. It was a lesson I had to learn the hard way.

Restaurant food can be eaten (and yes... even enjoyed) if you keep these tips in mind.

1. **Do some spying before going into battle.** Before the days of the Internet this would have required hiding in the restaurant's kitchen behind a pile of dirty dishes somewhere. This kind of sleuthing is no longer necessary. Simply take a few minutes and check out the restaurant's website before ordering. A majority of restaurants have posted their menus online, and many of them also include calorie information. Know what you are going to order in advance and stick to it.

2. **It is OK to say "no, thanks" when your waiter or waitress tries to hand you a menu.** At some point during the last century a clever restaurant owner discovered the power of putting pictures of food on the menu. Its purpose is to tempt you and (of course) increase the size of your bill. Unfortunately it can also increase the size of your waistline. If seeing pictures of onion rings and brownie sundaes makes you light-headed, tell your server that you don't need to see a menu. You already know what you'd like to order (because you did some menu spying ahead of time). You know exactly which dishes will fit into your daily calorie goal.

3. **Be careful in smaller, locally owned restaurants.** This final tip for eating out makes me sad. I am a *big* fan of family-owned businesses, and that includes restaurants. I have fond memories of my Saturday lunches and the awesome grilled cheese sandwiches at the soda fountain in my hometown. Mom-and-pop places are a personal favorite of mine.

And even with all this nostalgia, these local land-marks are the most dangerous restaurants when you are counting calories. The problem? Many of these places don't provide nutritional information about their foods. They can't tell you the calories in each dish because they don't *know* the actual number. A chicken sandwich may seem like a smart choice until it arrives at your table. Maybe it was described on the menu as grilled, but it will still pack a calorie punch when the lean bird is buried under a thick slice of bread, cheese, mayo, and bacon.

WEIGHING IN ON MOM-AND-POP RESTAURANTS

"Eat to live, but don't live to eat." These deep words of wisdom aren't mine. They actual originate from a quote by Socrates: "Worthless people live only to eat and drink; people of worth eat and drink only to live."[2] On the surface it seems like a healthy way to approach the dinner table. Humans would eat only the protein, fiber, vitamins, and minerals required to power our bodies through life. Our intake of food becomes a bodily function as devoid of emotion as breathing. We are simply filling up our tank, and any gas station will do.

I think the "eat to live and not live to eat" idea from Socrates is 50 percent right. I've put my own twist on this ancient diet slogan, and I'm dedicating it to all the mom-and-pop restaurants out there with hot coffee and laminated menus. I now present Linda's half-stolen philosophy on a healthy diet: love to eat but love God more.

I debated using the word *love* and almost took it out several times. Love is our fallback feeling to describe everything from our devotion to the Lord to our favorite jeans at the mall. America has worn out those four, tired letters. But after some thought I believe I can defend my use of the word.

When I weighed three hundred pounds, I was sure that a love

for food was my biggest problem. It seemed logical that a morbidly obese person would be the president of the "Hooray for Food" fan club; logical, but wrong. I actually hated food on most days. I was its slave. My cravings for fat and sugar were so intense that everything else in my life lost its flavor.

It wasn't just the time I spent putting food into my mouth. I wasted hundreds of hours thinking about food, sitting in drive-through lanes, and wishing I wasn't obese. There is no doubt that "fruits, grains, and the fatted calf" are gifts from the Lord. I got into trouble because these gifts *became* my Lord. I put food first. It didn't make me worthless (I don't care what Socrates said), but it did leave me feeling powerless.

So what is the alternative? Should our dinner be demoted to the status of a nine-volt battery? I believe that a healthy relationship with food starts with an understanding that our meals will always be more than just potential energy. There are sensations, emotions, and memories at the end of our forks. What is our very first "group" activity at birth? Eating. How did the father celebrate the return of his prodigal son? With eating. How do we mark birthdays, anniversaries, graduations, and even funerals? By eating.

My grandmother passed away a few years ago, and a tiny church in Higbee, Missouri, fed nearly fifty people after the services (even though no one in my family attends this church or has ever put money in its collection plate). The very definition of love is giving people what they need most when they deserve it the least. This church got it. These men and women understood that food is more than just protein, carbs, and fat. It carries emotion and offers comfort.

In this chapter we looked at how important it is to plan your meals ahead of time and know the estimated calories for each dish when you eat away from home. It is an essential rule for getting to and staying at a healthy weight. And like all good rules, sometimes it needs to be broken. Did the Higbee church have a website giving the nutritional information for the food it served? No. Did the ladies in the kitchen know how many calories were in every casserole dish? Probably not. Did I grab a plate and eat with my family after my grandmother's funeral? Absolutely.

For a healthy weight plan to be successful, it must be flexible enough to bend without breaking. It must accommodate those times in life when you just need to sit down with family and friends and enjoy a meal together. I have no idea how many calories I ate after my grandmother's funeral, and that's OK. You don't have to sneak away and eat raw vegetables in the car to protect your weight-loss plan. Here are some tips to help you build a plate that you can enjoy without guilt.

1. The 5 percent blind rule

When you don't have specific nutrition and calorie information for the plate of food in front of you, it is what I call a "blind" meal. I have some good news and some bad news about these mystery dishes. The good news? It is almost impossible to do permanent damage to a diet plan by eating just one high-calorie meal. The bad news? You will have "pound problems" if your information-poor/calorie-rich meals become a daily habit.

Life is sometimes messy and hectic. You will be in situations where you just don't know how many calories are on your plate. Work to keep your "blind" meals at 5 percent of your total meals consumed. That is approximately one meal a week if you eat breakfast, lunch, and dinner every day. If your friends want to try the local diner's chicken fried steak on a Friday night or if your mom is gathering everyone together for a big Sunday lunch, keep your other meals for the week within your daily calorie goals.

2. Watch out for too much BS (butter, batter, sauce, starch, and sugar)

If you've struggled with your weight for years, this isn't a news flash. Foods that are battered and fried, foods that are covered in a buttery or cheesy sauce, and foods with a lot of sugars and starches are higher in calories. Unfortunately, this BS rule even applies at church dinners. The key is to keep the foods you love and pass on the foods you only like. I will eat macaroni and cheese without complaining, but I love a good homemade roll with butter. I say "no, thanks" to the mac and cheese, and "oh, yeah" to the bread.

3. Blind doesn't mean mute

You may not know how many calories are on the menu at your favorite restaurant, but you can still customize your meal. Most locally owned establishments value your business enough to be flexible in the kitchen. And because these restaurants are small, your conversation doesn't have to stop with your server. Talk directly to the manager or the cook behind the grill. Be polite, but explain that you are trying to eat lighter for health reasons. If they can put grilled chicken on a salad, they can put it on a sandwich (even if the only chicken sandwich offered on the menu is breaded and fried). Spend your precious dollars with restaurants that are cheerfully willing to accommodate your needs.

A quick note to our local restaurants: I'm sure you've noticed that we, your devoted customers, are taking more space in the booth than we did twenty years ago. We need your help, and all it requires is creativity and a little experimentation. Our goal isn't to take over your entire menu. We just have some questions for you to think about: Can you substitute a few ingredients and make a lighter version of your popular items? Could we have smaller portions without being sent to the kid's menu? Could you give us nutritional information on a few dishes that have five hundred calories or less? On behalf of everyone who wants to live at a healthy weight, I can tell you that we miss eating in your restaurant. We'd like to make room for you at our table.

Your Weight Loss on Holiday

I felt hunted in the fall of 2007. It was deer season, but I wasn't afraid of Browning rifles, orange vests, or doe urine. In my opinion that was Bambi's problem. I had something more menacing in my own bathroom, and urine wasn't any part of it.

According to the calendar I was approaching my first holiday season on a diet plan. It can be a time of dread for anyone who doesn't want to "undo" weeks of tough weight-loss work. In 2007 my scale and I had formed an uneasy alliance, and I'd lost about forty pounds. But could that relationship continue through the Christmas eating season? Would the scale become the Grinch that steals my holiday joy? And how much weight will I gain if too many sugar plums dance in my mouth?

I didn't want to live the next six weeks running away from food. The angels outside of Bethlehem said, "Fear not!" I agreed. I had to find a way to enjoy holiday eating without worrying about my waistline or feeling guilty every time I sampled a piece of Christmas candy. I made a decision to relax my goal of losing one or two pounds per week, but I also refused to gain pounds between Thanksgiving and New Year's Day. What I needed was a "holiday hold."

It was a good name for my plan because I was constantly telling myself to "just hold on" when I was in a situation with too many tempting foods. I had more than a few unhealthy habits in my past—almost unconscious behaviors that I had developed after thirty-nine Christmas seasons of eating, drinking, and making merry. They had to be identified and confronted if I wanted to stay friends with my scale.

The Ghost of Christmas Eating Past

When I honestly examined my pattern of holiday snacking, grazing, and gorging, I found some strange reasons for overeating. Some of these habits may be haunting your table too:

1. **I ate food at parties and dinners that didn't taste good.** I was raised to clean my plate, but that "cleaning" often meant choking down barely tolerable

dishes. Isn't it sad to gain weight during the holiday season on food items that aren't even worth the calories that are in them?

2. **I ate food at parties and dinners to make other people feel good.** Please don't misunderstand me. I think it is great to encourage the budding chefs around you, but I didn't need to single-handedly be the taste tester for every cook in the room. And could I even call it taste testing when I ate two or three portions of every item?

3. **I kept the celebration going when I ate alone.** This is where the majority of my extra holiday calories came from. I used the Christmas season and my busy schedule as an excuse to add high-fat/high-sugar snacks, appetizers, and desserts into my already high-calorie diet. What could be more festive after a long day of shopping than a pie served in a cardboard box or an eggnog-flavored shake served through a drive-through window?

I wish the Ghost of Christmas Eating Past could report that calories take a holiday vacation, but they add up the same way in December as they do during the month of January. One pound of body fat is approximately 3,500 extra calories. My challenge in 2007 was how to track my calories when so many events and parties involved "blind eating." I needed a way to make smart choices when no one (including the cooks) could tell me how many calories were in their holiday treats.

The Ghost of Christmas Eating Present

Call it luck (or more likely a blessing straight from the Lord), but I made it through the 2007 holiday season without gaining weight and without hiding from holiday parties. It felt like a Christmas miracle. I didn't realize it at the time, but I was developing some strategies that I continue to use today when confronted with a buffet of mystery dishes. Take these tips to your next party:

1. Go heavy on the fruits and veggies.

I fill at least 60 percent of my plate with these colorful choices and give meats and carbohydrates the remaining 40 percent. But before you start piling on the creamed corn and cranberry sauce, I need to warn you that not all fruits and vegetables deserve majority status on your plate.

Corn isn't a vegetable. It is actually a grain and must be treated like a starch. Look for fruits and vegetables that are as close to their "roots" as possible. For example, cranberries shouldn't wiggle, and they don't naturally grow in the shape of an aluminum can. Broccoli isn't harvested wrapped in a blanket of cheddar cheese, and lettuce shouldn't look like a flotation device in a pool of ranch dressing. Finally, remember that the word *casserole* will toss a veggie into the starch category pretty quick.

It may have started its life as a fruit or vegetable, but could the average five-year-old identify it anymore? If the answer is no, confine it to the smaller 40 percent of your plate.

2. Turn on your BS detector (butter, batter, starch, sauce and sugar).

I would be a hypocrite if I told you to never eat a buttered roll, a Christmas cookie, or a batter-dipped piece of meat. I still eat these things, but only if they taste amazing. Be picky, and be aware that these food items will be higher in calories than our "un-messed-with" fruits and vegetables. Keep your portion sizes small, and remember they should fill 40 percent of the space on your plate or less. (Notice I am using the word "plate" here and not the word "platter." Don't put your food on any object that could double as a sled.)

3. Plan for parties ahead of time.

If you know your company's Christmas dinner will be a delicious array of tempting foods, eat a light breakfast and lunch. This is not the same thing as skipping breakfast or lunch. I repeat, do not skip meals in preparation for a big dinner. This strategy will backfire, make your blood sugar go crazy, and actually lead to overeating. About an hour before an event, I eat a 100- to 150-calorie snack with some good fiber or lean protein. It is just enough food to keep me from flirting with too many gingerbread men at the party.

The Ghost of Christmas Eating Future

I'm hesitating here because I don't want my good news to lead you into bad choices. When asked how much weight the average American gains between Thanksgiving and Christmas, most people estimate between five and ten pounds. It is actually one pound. According to a study reported by the National Institute of Health, fewer than 10 percent of us gain more than five pounds over the holiday season.[3]

Dr. Jack Yanovski, the principal study investigator for the National Institute of Child Health and Human Development, said "overweight and obese volunteers were more likely to gain five pounds than were those who were not overweight, which suggests that the holiday season may present special risks for those who are already overweight."[4]

The report also showed that once Americans put on a few holiday pounds, it rarely comes off.[5] Our "overly festive" eating choices today can lead to future problems with obesity. If you gain just one yearly "Christmas pound" beginning at the age of twenty, you will be thirty pounds overweight by the age of fifty. Sometimes the simple math problems are the most painful to solve!

WHEN YOU FEEL LIKE YOU'VE BLOWN IT

It's time once again to separate firm facts from fat fiction—one of my favorite things to do! We've examined the lies of obesity.

Unfortunately there is another set of "myths" that will creep up once you start a weight-loss plan. They may seem innocent enough on the surface, perhaps even noble. Don't be deceived. These lies can leave you feeling discouraged if you don't expose them for what they are. Be on the lookout for my three flabby fibs.

Flabby Fib One: If I am faithful to my weight-loss plan, I will lose pounds every week.

The Truth: Humans are wonderfully made, but we are not machines. On average I lost 1.5 pounds each week during my 155-pound weight loss. The important concept here is "average." If you want evidence proving how complex our bodies can be (especially the body of a woman), start a weight-loss program! There were several frustrating weeks when I didn't lose a single pound even after diligently counting my calories. I eventually figured out that this wasn't a battle against my scale. It was a war against my calendar, and patience had to be my weapon.

Even five years later I still remember how fragile my faith was during the initial weeks of my weight loss. It hurt *a lot* when it didn't seem I was making any progress. I would start to have these thoughts around day twelve of the standoff between my calendar and me: "What's the use? I knew this wouldn't work. I might as well go back to eating like I did before and forget about losing weight. I don't need all this stress."

When you start to feel like quitting, recognize this spot in the road for what it really is. You've reached an intersection. You can turn away from your healthy path or say a prayer, take a deep breath, and keep traveling forward. Your ultimate victory over obesity will come down to these critical moments of faith. It is at this fork in the road where so many weight-loss plans die. Your decision will mean everything. Time and time again I had to ask the Lord for strength and push through my doubts. I was often rewarded with a two- or three-pound drop on the scale just a few days later.

Flabby Fib Two: Exercise is easy for healthy people. They like it.

The Truth: I generally exercise five days out of seven. That adds up to be 260 workouts a year. And even with all that sweat, there are still days when I would rather find a comfortable couch and put my feet up. I've asked personal trainers, marathon runners, and athletes if they also have days where their calendar says work out and their brain says veg out. They do. That is when the experts recommend some mental negotiations.

Agree in your mind to exercise, but go with half of the time or distance you had originally planned. After several weeks getting even a small amount of daily exercise can add up to lost pounds and a healthier heart. When I finish a walk or a trip to the gym, I am always glad I made the effort. Remember this feeling when you are in "negotiations" with your brain.

Flabby Fib Three: I've eaten nothing but junk all day, and now my diet is dead.

The Truth: Remember what you've learned so far. One pound of weight gain is approximately 3,500 extra calories. These are calories above the number needed by your body to power you through the day and keep you alive. Unless you entered a pie-eating contest, the most you can gain after one "bad day" is probably a pound or two. Is it a setback? Yes, a small one. Does it have to be the end of your weight-loss plan? Absolutely not.

There is, however, some strange thinking that can occur *after* our high-calorie day, and it's where the real danger lies. We make a conscious choice to turn a "bad day" into a "bad week." This is a common attitude during the holiday season, and I've been guilty of this destructive pattern more than a few times.

Even if these decisions don't come straight from the devil, I think they must make him giggle a little. Here is the gist of how I would justify this in my head: "I ate terribly yesterday. I'm going to write off this whole week and start my diet again on Monday. It will be a fresh start." Dangerous thinking!

Although it may be hard to kill a weight-loss plan in just one day, you can do some weighty damage when it turns into several days of overeating. Let's be honest. You will probably fall off the wagon during your weight loss. I did more than once, and I still have days when I don't make the smartest food choices.

Before your feet hit the floor the next morning, get in touch with your inner Barney Fife and "nip it in the bud." Don't let a bad day turn into a bad week and beyond. A pound isn't too tough to lose, but shedding an extra ten pounds can mean a month or more of hard work. Nip those bad days in the bud, and wake up the next day back on your plan.

When I weighed three hundred pounds, I thought being a healthy size would require a tremendous sacrifice over a short period of time. My goal was to lose the weight as quickly as possible with starvation plans and excessive exercise. The reality of my weight loss ended up being something completely different. It was a long journey with tiny sacrifices that felt less like sacrifices every day. Through it I learned more about myself and my God than I ever could have imagined.

There is a verse in the Bible that reads, "Well done, good and faithful servant."[6] I've known that scripture since I was a little girl. It wasn't until my weight loss, however, that I understood how important the second adjective really is in that sentence. As imperfect humans being good in Master's eyes is...good. But when we combine good with faithful (a stubbornness to continue forward even after we fall), we become a tool that fits perfectly in the Lord's hands.

House Call With Nick Yphantides, MD

Question: In your book, *My Big Fat Greek Diet*, you are very honest about your love of restaurants...specifically fast food. Can that type of food be a part of someone's healthy weight loss?

Dr. Yphantides: Since fast food is so popular, any discussion on how to lose weight must address our eat-on-the-go culture. I don't think you have to give up fast food completely as you try to lose weight, but you certainly have to think intentionally each time you pull up to the drive-through lane. Here are a few ideas I give my patients:

1. Pay close attention to the lower-fat, lower-carbohydrate, lower-calorie items on the menu—and order those.

2. Make sure if it fries, it dies. Order broiled rather than breaded or deep-fried meat.

3. Stay away from bacon.

4. Don't say "cheese." It will generally add 40 percent more fat.

5. Hold the sauce or go with regular condiments such as mustard.

6. Say no to "supersized."

7. Remember that anything served with chicken (especially baked or broiled chicken) will have fewer calories than beef.

8. Go for the pita sandwiches

9. Order a salad with a low-cal or no-cal dressing.

10. Order with your mind and not your stomach. You have to keep your head when you step up to the counter. Order only what makes sense in regard to the number of calories that you can eat every day to maintain weight loss.

Chapter Eleven

GETTING TO YOUR GOAL WEIGHT
AND STAYING THERE

I'VE HAD A colorful and odd assortment of dieting attempts through the years. Some of them were actually healthy weight-loss plans, but I always put the pounds back on. If you've been overweight for any length of time, you probably have some diet "practice" in your past too.

My short list of failed weight-loss plans include:

1. Fen-Phen. This is a prescription no longer available because of claims that it can damage the heart.

2. Xenical (now sold over the counter as Alli). This is the weight-loss pill with all of the interesting side effects. It was the first time I ever heard the phrase "oily stools" in reference to the human body. A great day.

3. Slim Fast

4. Atkins

5. Richard Simmon's Deal-A-Meal. Remember that one?

6 Workout videos (some still in their original wrappers)

7. The Banana Diet. This is one I tried in college. You eat nothing but bananas for breakfast and lunch. If you can make it to the table, you are allowed a

sensible dinner in the evening. This diet will make you wish for oily stools or really any stools at all.

8. Three separate gym memberships (with very little attendance but some steep monthly fees)

9. A treadmill (that is now in my basement and makes a great coat rack)

10. A failed attempt to have gastric bypass surgery (my insurance company wouldn't pay for it)

So how should we look at these less-than-successful attempts? Are they failures? Are they messages from God that obesity is just our burden to bear? It's time to give ourselves a break. Or better yet, let's give ourselves a "brake" and think back to the first time we got behind the wheel of an automobile. Even after twenty-five years my memories of being a young driver aren't pretty.

I grew up in a rural area, but I didn't have the "driving the farm truck" experience that most teens had in Central Missouri. My driver's education car was a 1980 Ford LTD, and the instructor was the football coach at my high school. The entire semester felt like a disaster at the time. My ability to do push-ups improved (thanks, coach), but I still couldn't put on the brakes without giving everyone in the car whiplash. It was months before I could drive over the nearby Missouri River without getting light-headed and nauseous.

I often walked away from that Ford LTD embarrassed and discouraged. My passengers often stumbled away thankful to be alive. I wasn't able to hide my inability to keep a consistent speed, stay on the right side of the road, and avoid the potholes. Everyone knew I was struggling, and yet no one told me to quit. Even my poor football coach (who probably lost a head of hair that semester) never said, "Linda, I think it is God's will for you to remain a pedestrian for the rest of your life."

It was understood that we were mastering a new skill. It was understood that we wouldn't get it right the first time or even the tenth time. It was understood that making mistakes (and seeing our fellow classmates make mistakes) was important. Every time we swerved into a ditch or rolled backward in drive, we were learning what not to do. A student might forget the words in a driver's manual, but she will never forget the first time she had to steer her car out of the weeds. Those lessons stick.

It's time to stop being embarrassed and discouraged by our failures. If you have a long list of weight-loss attempts in your past, good for you! You now have some sharp tools in your bag that you will need going forward. Recognize these assets for what they are. Looking back at my twenty years of diets, I learned that:

1. **I must pay attention to nutritional information.** Just assuming that something is low in calories will get me in the weeds.

2. **The cravings for high-fat and high-sugar foods won't last forever.** For me, they lasted about six weeks. All of my weight-loss "failures" taught me to hang on tight to the wheel and keep driving past that forty-day mark. Eventually my stomach and my brain will sign a peace treaty and learn to play nice.

3. **Never, never go on a diet that requires eating a large number of bananas every day.**

Losing weight and maintaining a healthy size is a skill. Just like with driving a car, there are rules of the road. Do your best to learn these guidelines, but understand that putting the rules in your head doesn't replace testing them on hard pavement. After your first week you might get tired of paying so much attention to portion sizes. After your third week you might lose three pounds and gain one right back. After your fifth week you might start an exercise plan and let it go when your schedule gets too busy.

The world will call these attempts setbacks, but the world is wrong. It's a set-forward because you are now a smarter driver. You've seen the potholes, you've rolled backward in drive, and you've been in the weeds. I spent more than twenty years trying to steer out of the ditch. I can tell you that the lessons I learned were sometimes painful. But as long as you have the courage to keep moving forward, God can take your failures and struggles and give you wisdom and strength in return.

THE RIGHT REASON TO TAKE THE JOURNEY

Because of a passable alto voice I had the opportunity to witness the glory days of a church choir one summer in college. The volunteer director, a gray-haired lady who swayed when she played the organ, was passing the baton to a new music minister and his soprano wife. This couple was young, attractive, and brought our small congregation some ideas that were revolutionary at the time. Instead of singing with a traditional keyboard, we tried choral pieces with a full orchestra on cassette tape.

Side note: For those of you born after 1990, cassettes were plastic and about the size of an iPhone. But instead of holding thousands of songs, it could only store a few. It was fun to put your favorite tunes on a "mix tape" and give it to the person you were dating. The best part about owning a "mix" was that you could rip the tape out of the cassette after a bad breakup and the music would never play again. It was pretty symbolic stuff in 1987, but let's get back to the story.

Under the direction of this dynamic music minister, the choir doubled in size. People who had worn only bathrobes on a Sunday morning were putting on choir robes. We finally had enough men that we could tackle music with an intimidating "SATB" printed on the front cover. This choir was learning what it meant to make a joyful noise to the Lord in four-part harmony.

On the August weekend before I returned to Mizzou, we had

fifty people in the choir loft. Those were strong numbers in a church that averaged four hundred members at its Sunday services. I packed for college believing I had witnessed a mini-revival within this small congregation. I was only twenty years old and still had some things to learn about motivation.

The young minister received a job offer from a larger church in the fall of 1988. A larger church meant a larger music budget and a larger salary for his family. When I went home to attend the Christmas Eve services that year he and his soprano wife were gone. Also gone was the four-part harmony. The choir was down to its "pre-cassette" numbers and sang to the accompaniment of a gray-haired lady who swayed when she played the organ.

Maybe I'm just a music geek in my soul, but watching the choir that Christmas was disheartening. What had happened? How could the loss of two people do this much damage? Why were so many former choir members missing from the ranks? I squirmed in my pew and counted the minutes until I could question my mom (a much better alto than me) and get the inside scoop. She was one of the faithful who still wore the robes.

When worship gets worldly

There is no doubt that this church choir was worshipping as it grew under the direction of the young music minister. The problem was that many of its members weren't worshipping God. They had a dynamic and energetic leader in front of them—someone they could see and touch. It was his encouragement and approval that motivated the singers to attend rehearsals, pick up a hymnal, and do the work required to be successful. When he was gone, so was their reason for worship. I'm sure I wasn't the only person to leave that Christmas Eve service wondering what happened.

It was easy for me at the age of twenty to judge this choir for its misguided motivations. Twenty-five years later I understand that the log in my eye makes it hard for me to see the speck in someone else's. We are all guilty of world worship. It can lift us high. But because it is built on sand, there is no lasting foundation. It doesn't sustain us. We limp away battered, broken, and asking, "What happened?" when we crash back to the ground.

When weight loss gets worldly

After stepping on the bathroom scale, the "what happened?" question is often the first thing out of our mouths (after a few colorful expletives). It has happened again. The weight-loss plan that seemed so promising isn't working. This disappointment is a constant companion for yo-yo dieters. We gain and lose the same pounds over and over again...even after our promises that this time the weight is going to stay off for good.

Our motivations for weight loss—the incentives that carried us in the beginning—now seem weak in the face of daily food temptations. The search begins for another diet plan that guarantees lasting results. At some point during this never-ending cycle we need to ask ourselves this question, "Is our weight-loss plan at fault, or could it be that our motivations to lose weight are built on sand?"

There are a few good reasons to lose weight and a million bad ones. These negative motivators generally fall under three categories:

1. Because we want to please another person

For several years after the Christmas Eve service of 1988 I wondered about those missing church choir members. Where they able to find another dynamic leader to inspire them? How many times has their worship of a human (rather than the Lord) let them down? Are they still singing?

People, even people with the best of intentions, will eventually disappoint us. The choir director we followed was attractive, energetic, and passionate about his work. He stood in front of us every week to encourage worship—not to be the reason for our worship. Like all humans, his power to influence was temporary. He left us. And for many of the choir members so did their reasons for singing. They had motivations built on sand.

2. Because we believe that achieving a diet goal is the key to happiness

Living at a healthy weight allows your body to do the work God had planned for you from the moment you were conceived. If you believe a number on a scale or a size printed inside your jeans will bring you happiness, get ready for a crash. You are standing on sand.

Pounds and proportions are cold numbers. They won't give your life a purpose, and they won't make this planet a better place to live after you are gone. The sweat required in order to lose weight ultimately gives us the energy needed to sweat in the service of others. This is where the real joy of weight loss is found.

3. Because we equate being thinner with being valued

This is a nasty one. It's true that some shallow humans will base your worthiness as a person on your weight. If the two misguided motivators I listed above are resting on sand, this one is built on quicksand.

I think it is interesting to look at this idea of "value" from the Lord's perspective. He has seen countless cultures rise and fall. Some valued "fat" as a sign of prosperity. It was evidence that your family was blessed with an abundance of food. On the other hand, a "skinny" body was proof that your family was struggling to provide. A pleasantly plump appearance was valued within these societies.

Even with so many changing standards about weight, it is ultimately the Lord's opinion that matters. It is the one thing that is constant and unchanging. God tells us to treat our bodies like a temple. He doesn't care about some random number on a scale, but He does care if we worship the wrong things, trash the temple, and leave french fry wrappers under the pews.

I'VE LOST THE WEIGHT. NOW WHAT?

I am a "before and after" photo junkie. I've been that way my whole life. Even when I weighed three hundred pounds, I would grab some snacks, flop down on the couch, and watch weight-loss info-mercials just to see the before and after pictures. My dream was that someday I would find more willpower, find the right diet, or find a magic pill that would make my fat melt away.

I always thought, "Good grief, we can put a man on the moon. Can't somebody invent an easy solution for weight loss? I've been waiting twenty years. I know I will be *so* happy once I finally get thin. After picture, here I come."

It doesn't seem to matter if we need to lose fifteen pounds or one hundred fifty pounds. We all imagine that day when we finally reach our ideal weight. Our hair will be thicker. Our teeth will be whiter. Our jokes will be funnier. Who knows? Maybe birds will stop leaving little gifts on our cars.

I don't think there is anything wrong with having a picture of how life will be different at a smaller size. My ultimate dream was to shop in a store with "regular" sizes and actually be able to zip my pants. A fine goal to have! And when we reach our final desti-nation, we envision a level of joy and satisfaction that can be very motivating during our journey. It can also be very dangerous once we achieve our goal.

THE CHRISTMAS MORNING CRASH

You've spent weeks dreaming and scheming. It all comes down to this one, wonderful moment when you see what is waiting for you under the Christmas tree. In 1976 my hopes were riding high on the Easy Bake Oven. I imagined making a veritable cornucopia of desserts...all with the cooking power of an ordinary light bulb. No more waiting for my mom to whip up treats. I would run my own bakery in my bedroom! (A foreshadow of future weight issues? Maybe.)

- **At 6:30 a.m.** on that Christmas morning, I was the happiest child in Randolph County, Missouri. The Easy Bake Oven was mine and the first cake was in the oven.

- **At 9:30 a.m.** I was coming down from a sugar high and realizing I had baked every packet of cake mix in the box. The party was over. My dream of the perfect Christmas present wasn't as sweet as I imagined it would be.

- **At 11:00 a.m.** I started dreaming about what Santa could bring next year.

I hope I've matured since that Christmas morning in 1976, but I still have moments when I look to the world for contentment. We all do. It starts with those famous six words. "I would be happy if only..." Plug in your own answer.

I have a spoiler alert for everyone holding this book who wants to lose weight and reach that "after picture" moment. It won't live up to the hype. Being thinner (in and of itself) won't bring you lasting joy. I thank God for that. Imagine how shallow our lives would be if we could achieve eternal contentment through a number on a scale...if our only goal was to present the "perfect" physical picture to the world. It makes me tired just thinking about it.

Because we are made in the image of the Lord, we are more complex than that. And because we *aren't* Lord, our complexity can trip us up. It's the dreaded feeling of "This is it? This is what I worked so hard for?" We can be itchy, restless people just days after we achieve a victory. I think this is why most fairy tales wrap up the story with "and they lived happily ever after." We don't really want to see the next chapter.

I have a strange confession. Maybe it's my overactive maternal instinct, but I worry about star athletes when they finally win the "big game." After years of hitting tennis balls, she finally lifts the

Wimbledon cup above her head. After years of tossing a football through a tire, he finally throws the winning touchdown in the fourth quarter of the Super Bowl.

We sit on our couches and watch the media hype that immediately follows these gifted athletes. We think to ourselves, "It would be great to be them." We don't see the natural letdown that follows these victories until pictures (such as the one of Olympic swimmer Michael Phelps with a bong) hit the tabloids. We don't see that moment when an athlete says to himself, "So, this is what it feels like to be a champion. Is this as good as it gets?"

After any long journey the kid inside each one of us will experience a "Christmas morning crash." You finally have within your hands that thing you've only dreamed of, and the "wow" factor just isn't there. It's how you respond to this feeling that means everything. *Everything.* It's the difference between the 90 percent of dieters who will put the weight back on and the 10 percent who will maintain a healthy size.

When I was obese, I wasn't the only one with an after photo in mind. God had some plans for me that went way beyond the three-hundred-pound body that the world could see on the outside. When I finally hit my weight-loss goal in 2009, these plans ended up being the perfect cure for my own "Christmas morning crash."

Take your "OK, what now?" questions to God. He probably has a few things to say. We pay so much attention to the external, but the Lord knows what we can accomplish for the eternal. We can get too focused on food. The Lord wants us to taste freedom. We get obsessed with "will" power. God can see how much more is possible if I we simply pray for "Thy will" to be done.

One hundred fifty-five pounds lighter, I'm still learning. There are days when I don't make the smartest food choices. There are weather forecasts that keep me from exercise. There are dark moments when I mourn all of the years I wasted on my obesity...time I spent feeling guilty about the food I ate, wishing I were thinner, hating the way that I looked. It's OK. We have a Savior, and our best after picture is still to come.

House Call With Rita Hancock, MD

Question: In order to stop my twenty-year cycle of losing weight and gaining it right back, I had to pay more attention to the places I go and the people I spent time with. How important is the environment around us?

Dr. Hancock: Your environment is extremely important. You can't just go with the flow of the world, or you might be unduly influenced by other people's negativity, emotional conflict, poor attitudes, and bad habits (such as overvaluing food and overeating), and strife. I once heard a preacher say it's as if we have "emotional Wi-Fi." We pick up emotional strife from the people around us. In turn I believe those negative emotions can lead us to stress eat if we're prone to eating for emotional reasons.

You're better off choosing to hang around people who love God and who have good health habits rather than give yourself over to the thoughts and attitudes of people who are bad for you.

Chapter Twelve

NAGGING YOU ONE MORE TIME

You WIN. I can't take the peer pressure anymore. I've been strong for several pages, but I'm waving the white flag of surrender. It's meal plan time.

If you've read every chapter of this book, you know I didn't provided you with a meal plan of what I specifically ate during my weight loss. It's not that I'm trying to be sneaky or secretive about the details. I wasn't on the Andrew Zimmern *Bizarre Foods* diet. (If you've never watched this show on the Travel Channel, you've missed Andrew eat culinary treats such as a jellied moose nose, teriyaki cockroaches, and a llama's brain. Yum!)

The foods I ate during my weight loss were far less bizarre than Andrew's TV diet. And even with my more traditional menu, I understand that a dish I rank as "delicious" may be given a "disgusting" score by you. Taste buds are as personalized as a fingerprint.

So before I share a day in the life of my weight-loss plate, you must swear an oath and promise you won't get snarky with me if:

1. **Your doctor vetoes this menu for health reasons** (that is, you have food allergies, a gluten intolerance, issues with sodium, and so on).

2. **You are a vegetarian, vegan, or eat only raw foods** (foods with an internal temperature of 118 degrees Fahrenheit or less).

3. You have diet restrictions for religious reasons
(or you believe that vegetables are nothing more than weeds planted by the devil).

I am giving you a 1,500-calorie day using common, name-brand items that can be found in most supermarkets. The generic or "store brand" versions of these items are often less expensive. Read the labels to check their calorie per serving information. It might pay to shop around.

If you weigh three hundred fifty pounds and work as a lumberjack, you will need more food than what I've put on my plate below. That's OK. I think you will be pleasantly surprised at how many calories you can eat every day and still lose weight.

I know. I've stalled long enough. After several pages of anticipation, I present to you...

A RELUCTANT MEAL PLAN—1,500-CALORIE DAY

Breakfast

2 medium eggs scrambled with ¼ cup Kraft
    2 percent shredded cheddar cheese and a little salt/pepper
1 Sara Lee whole-grain English muffin (to hold all the eggy-cheesy goodness)
1 small apple
Any noncalorie beverage (water, black coffee, green tea, and the like)
Total approximate breakfast calories: 406

Lunch

2 tablespoons creamy Jif peanut butter on two slices of Wonder Light Wheat bread
1 cup sliced cucumbers

½ cup fresh blueberries

1 ounce Rold Gold pretzel twists

Any noncalorie beverage

Total approximate lunch calories: 443

Dinner

1 3-ounce flank steak

12 steamed green beans (about 4 inches long)

1 medium baked potato with the skin on (no more than 3.5 inches in diameter)

2 tablespoons reduced-fat sour cream and salt/pepper to taste

Any noncalorie beverage

Total approximate dinner calories: 272

Snacks (spread throughout the day or added to any meal)

2 cups shredded romaine lettuce with 3 ounces lean turkey and 2 tablespoons Kraft Light Done Right Zesty Italian Dressing

1 6-ounce serving of Dannon Light & Fit Strawberry Yogurt

1 serving of Pop Secret's 100-calorie popcorn

Water, water, and water

Total approximate snack calories: 309

If you are doing the math, all of this food is approximately 1,430 calories. You could add three Hershey's Kisses to get even closer to 1,500 calories. And in the spirit of full disclosure, I admit that this menu is not a completely perfect one...if such a thing even exists. I wanted to give you a real picture of what I ate during my weight loss, but here are some possible improvements.

I am missing beans (which I like) and fish (which I generally don't like to eat). I have included a steak on my dinner menu, but I ate red meat only about three times a week. I also have pretzels, popcorn, and Hershey's Kisses on my plate because they are fun. While these "junk foods" may lack nutrition, I would argue that they bring valuable emotional benefits to the table.

Snacks gave my weight-loss menu some vitamin S. It was "sanity" during my diet. For twenty years I tried plans with weird foods or foods in weird amounts (like nothing but bananas for breakfast and lunch). The result? I would feel weird and want to quit after the first day. The plate that finally worked for me felt so normal that I didn't want to quit. It was reasonably balanced, allowed me to eat all day long, and helped me stay full. If it included a few splurges from time to time, so be it.

Eat foods you enjoy. It sounds like common sense, but you never want to choke down someone else's menu simply because it is low in calories. Use the tools in this book and take the time to develop your own plate of sanity. Need some yummy ideas? Check out my blog at www.theskinnybudgetdiet.com and find lighter versions of your favorite comfort foods.

A Lighter Bucket List

Before I let you go, we need to talk about your future. You can have a seven-figure income, live in a five-thousand-square-foot house, and have an IQ of 162. But unless God has other plans, there is only one number that really matters. Your life here on this earth is 100 percent fatal. Do you have things you want to accomplish before you die? Have you made your bucket list?

I've been secretly peeking into the "pre-kicked buckets" of family, friends, and absolute strangers. Some popular goals include swimming with dolphins, learning to play a musical instrument, and traveling to an exotic location. I thought participating in the annual Cheese-Rolling Festival at Cooper's Hill in Gloucestershire was a fun idea. One guy wants to name a future son or daughter after the place where the child is conceived. I really hope this man doesn't live in Boring, Oregon, or Embarrass, Minnesota. Junior high is tough enough if your first name is simply John.

I was surprised how many people put "lose weight" on their bucket lists. Even when I was three hundred–plus pounds, burning extra fat wasn't glamorous enough to make my top ten list of goals. Where is the wow factor? Vowing to diet sounded about as exciting to me as pledging to clean the garage or floss my teeth more often. I wanted to throw a coin in the Trevi Fountain, climb the Spanish Steps, and walk the streets of Rome, not count calories, climb a StairMaster, and walk around the city park with my dog.

If you are morbidly obese or just need to lose twenty pounds, I think it is OK if weight loss isn't on your bucket list. A smaller body can't stand alone as a life goal. It is simply a means to an end...a vehicle to move you toward the goals that really matter. Save the valuable space on your bucket list for adventures that take your breath away, but understand that the list now comes with a three-word preamble. Get healthy first.

I always wanted to travel to Europe. My body was too large to fit in an airplane seat. I wanted to scale the Spanish Steps (138 of them in all). My knees would have been screaming before I reached the halfway point. I wanted to stroll through the streets of Rome. The discomfort of feeling my thighs rub together would have sent me back to the hotel in less than thirty minutes.

Whenever I dreamed of places I could see with my husband or the activities that I could share with my sons, it was quickly followed by this depressing question: "You have big ideas, but can your big body pull it off?" In order to keep up with the mobile men in my family, I struggled to move while carrying the equivalent of another woman on my back. This 155-pound person stayed with me and never took a vacation just because I took a vacation.

I had an unwanted guest every time I walked down the street, rode a bike, climbed into a canoe, or splashed in the ocean. This extra person and I were kicked off of roller coasters and told that we were too heavy to go on a long trail ride. (Quarter horses were forced to organize a union to keep my oversized rear out of the saddle.) Most of the activities that stayed on my bucket list came with the disclaimer that a large dose of pain reliever would be required. It sucked the fun out of everything but the most sedentary of ideas.

As my body got bigger, my "must do" list of adventures got smaller. It was such a slow process that I didn't realize what was happening. The extra pounds were not only smothering my body but burying my dreams as well. By the time my scale passed the three hundred mark, all that I had left was joining a book club and singing the karaoke version of "You've Lost That Loving Feeling" to an uncomfortable crowd.

It was a sad place to be. Thankfully it was also a fixable place to be. If you are obese and your bucket list looks like the property of someone twice your age, I have some good news. My goals came alive when my body came alive. Yours will too. During the twenty months of my weight loss, questions evolved into statements. "Can my big body pull this off?" became "I think my smaller body can pull this off."

Your bucket list can be a powerful tool during your weight loss. It took me from Disney World to rafting class four rapids on the Pigeon River in Tennessee. Here's how to get the most out of your bucket:

1. **Organize your list of goals.** Put the least physical items at the top of the list and the more strenuous adventures near the bottom.

   Track how much money you are saving by dining out less and eating at home more. Set this money aside for the "bucket." By buying your food in bulk and having a meal plan, this fun slush fund will

grow quickly. Pay off your debts where needed, but
slowly put money aside for adventures.

Not to be morbid again, but I want your family
to have some great stories when they gather around
your deathbed. I don't think anyone will talk about
the beautiful couch you bought in the year 2014.
They will, however, remember the great adventure
of 2014 when everyone rode mules down into the
Grand Canyon. Focus more on sunsets and less on
stuff!

2. **Use this list to build your weight-loss rewards.**
My family spent a week riding roller coasters when
my scale finally fell below two hundred pounds.
Once I hit my final "resting" weight, quarter horses
could no longer turn me down, and my family rode
together through the Smoky Mountains.

My bucket list is still an active part of my "be healthier" journey.
In 2014 I will celebrate the five-year anniversary of reaching my
goal weight. I've seen the statistics. I know how difficult it can be
to keep the extra weight off and not become a yo-yo dieter. If I can
still walk the walk (in addition to talking the talk here with you),
I am going to Italy, and I will run up those 138 Spanish Steps. It
may be more of a slow jog once I get near the top, but I will do it.

Put this book down and make your own "God and I will do
this" list. Pray for the Lord's guidance, take the first small step,
and make it happen. When you finally kick the bucket (hopefully
many long years from now), I want your family and friends to tell
stories about your life that go long into the night.

Appendix

THE "SKINNY" ON THIS PLAN

A NOT-SO-SHOCKING NEWS FACT: If your body burns more calories than you eat, you will lose weight. One pound is approximately 3,500 calories. With the exception of a few rare medical conditions, this is true for all men and women.

Your daily calories requirements for your height, age, gender, and activity level are unique to you. It's also important to remember that your daily calorie requirements will change as your weight changes. When I weighed three hundred–plus pounds, I could eat 2,300 calories a day and lose two pounds each week. That number slowly fell as I lost weight.

QUICK-START SHOPPING GUIDE

Before you even step into the supermarket

1. **Get on the scale.** I know this might be painful if it has been a long time since you've seen that number, but you need to know what you weigh right now to set a reasonable weight-loss goal.

2. **Set an appointment with your doctor** and show up for the appointment. There are several important questions to ask your doctor, including: "Are there specific foods to include or avoid based on my health concerns or individual needs? What type of

exercise plan can I safely start? Do I need something low impact for my joints? What would be a healthy weight range for me?"

3. **Visit www.sparkpeople.com, www.livestrong .com/thedailyplate, or any of the free calorie-tracking websites available online.** Have a smart-phone? There are several outstanding tracking apps that you can download. I have myfitnesspal on my iPhone. Take ten minutes and set up a profile by entering your height, weight, age, gender, and activity level. Also enter how many pounds you would like to lose each week once you start a weight-loss plan. You will use this website to track your daily calories once your Skinny Budget Diet plan begins. Think of it as free training wheels!

4. **Track your calories for one week.** The best time to do this would be in the evening after your last meal or snack. Don't change your diet in any way at this point. Eat and drink what you would normally eat and drink, but pay attention to the cups, pounds, servings, etc. We need to know where we are before we can determine where we need to go.

5. **Track your exercise** (if any) that you've had during the day right along with your food. It will give you a more accurate reading of your net calories. Did you walk your dog for thirty minutes? Enter that information into your online tracker.

6. **Make a meal plan before you shop.** The goal is to eat more meals prepared at home and less drive-through, take-out, and delivery. This requires a plan. Use the free, online calorie-tracking website you've chosen to find specific information about

your favorite dishes. This is also a great place to see "lighter" alternatives to the foods you like. This meal plan should include breakfast, lunch, dinner, snacks, and beverages.

7. **Clean and restock your house.** Items you will need include measuring cups. storage containers, bags that zip (to put bulk items into individual servings), and a scale. Remove snacks from your kitchen that aren't on your approved list, and double-check your staples before you shop. In the beginning of your weight loss you want to remove as many excuses not to cook as possible.

8. **Check the grocery store circulars for bargains.** This is also the time when you will organize your coupons and decide if shopping at more than one store will save you money. Using the information in your meal plan, the items in your kitchen, and your knowledge of sale items from the circulars, write your shopping list.

9. **Schedule grocery shopping at your peak.** Pushing a "purpose driven" shopping cart will take energy. Schedule your trip at a point during the day when you have the most energy. Avoid times during the week when the stores are crowded. I also recommend wearing layers and comfortable shoes.

10. **Eat a "snack" before shopping that includes lean protein and/or fiber.** Also remember to shop alone or with another adult who is focused on reading labels and unit prices.

When you step into the supermarket

1. **Put nonperishable items in your cart first and finish with the refrigerated and frozen items.** You don't want to feel rushed because the cold items are sweating or melting.

2. **Take a water and bench break.** This requires paying attention to your body. If you are feeling tired, it can be tempting to throw "whatever" in your cart just to get out of the store. The Skinny Budget Diet is all about knowledge. We want to know the calories per serving and the unit price for every edible item that goes into our carts.

3. **Spend more time in the outer circle.** The outside edge of most supermarkets is where fresh vegetables, fruits, and meats are found.

4. **Chew sugarless gum while standing in the checkout line.** You know that grocery stores put candy and salty treats on both sides of the checkout lane. They understand that we are weak—a tired and hungry audience. To resist the temptation, put in a fresh stick of gum and have a snack waiting for you in the car.

5. **Watch the register closely.** According to research the prices scanned at the supermarket registers are incorrect. Sometimes the mistakes are in your favor but not always. The top offenders are sale items, produce, and foods that aren't prepackaged. Find a spot where you can see the price for each product scanned.

After you leave the supermarket

1. **Bag snacks immediately into one-serving portions when you get home.** It is dangerous to leave food (especially snack foods) in their bulk, oversized packages. We can't save this job for "later" because the overeating risks are too high. Kick off your shoes, put on some music, and spend some time in your kitchen.

2. **Involve the whole family.** I don't recommend grocery shopping with children, but this is a great time to get them involved. With clean hands grab the measuring cups, a pile of sandwich or snack bags, and create a snack assembly line. Ideal foods for grab-and-go snacks are grapes, carrots, strawberries, nuts, cookies (if the calories are right), cereal, and trail mix.

3. **Be meticulous.** Read the nutritional information and understand the calories and the serving sizes. Measuring is crucial in the beginning of your weight-loss program in order to learn what a portion size actually looks like. These are your training wheels. They will come off as you lose weight and as your cravings diminish.

You will not count calories for the rest of your life. I was able to take the training wheels off of my weight-loss plan after twenty months of tracking and measuring. Depending on how many pounds you need to lose, you could be riding "solo" in even less time. Our ultimate goal is to have a relationship with food that is the way God intended, as healthy and natural as breathing.

NOTES

INTRODUCTION
LIVING HIGH ON THE HOG

1. Luke 16:10, KJV.

CHAPTER ONE
WASTING TIME ON A GROWING WAIST

1. Matthew 17:20.
2. See Jeremiah 29:11.

CHAPTER TWO
SEPARATING THE FACTS FROM FAT FICTION

1. Centers for Disease Control and Prevention, "Losing Weight," http://www.cdc gov/healthyweight/losing_weight/index.html (accessed September 13, 2012)

2. T. Pischon, H. Boeing, K. Hoffmann, et. al., "General and Abdominal Adiposity and Risk of Death in Europe" *The New England Journal of Medicine* 359, no. 20 (November 13, 2008): 2105–2120; http://www.nejm.org/doi/pdf/10.1056/NEJMoa0801891 (accessed September 7, 2012).

3. *ACE Personal Trainer Manual: The Ultimate Resource for Fitness Professionals*, 3rd edition (San Diego, CA: American Council on Exercise, 2003).

4. See Psalm 139:14.

CHAPTER THREE
COUNTING AND CLEANING

1. James Norman, "Hypothyroidism: Too Little Thyroid Hormone http://www.endocrineweb.com/conditions/thyroid/hypothyroidism-too-little-thyroid-hormone (accessed September 13, 2012).

2. Elizabeth Mendes, "Six in 10 Overweight or Obese in U.S., More in '09 Than in '08," Gallup Wellbeing, February 9, 2010, http://www.gallup.com/poll/125741/Six-Overweight-Obese.aspx (accessed September 13, 2012).

3. William Bennett and Joel Gurin, *The Dieter's Dilemma* (New York: Basic Books, 1982).

4. Kathleen Zelman, "The Real Truth About Belly Fat," UnitedHealthcare, http://tinyurl.com/d3pfclx (accessed September 13, 2012).

5. Heather I. Katcher, Richard S. Legro, Allen R. Kunselman, et. al., "The Effects of a Whole Grain–Enriched Hypocaloric Diet on Cardiovascular Disease Risk Factors in Men and Women With Metabolic Syndrome," *American Journal of Clinical Nutrition* 87, no. 1 (January 2008): 79–90.

6. Colette Bouchez, "9 Surprising Facts About Your Stomach," WebMD, http://women.webmd.com/pharmacist-11/stomach-problems (accessed September 10, 2012).

7. Ibid.

8. Elaine Magee, "The Facts About Food Cravings," WebMD, http://www.webmd.com/diet/features/the-facts-about-food-cravings (accessed September 13, 2012).

9. Ibid.

10. M.F. Dallman, N. Pecoraro, S.F. Akana, et. al., "Chronic Stress and Obesity: A New View of 'Comfort Food,'" *Proceedings of the National Academy of Sciences* 100, no. 20 (September 30, 2003).

11. Magee, "The Facts About Food Cravings."

12. Center for Disease Control and Prevention, "Body Measurements," http://www.cdc.gov/nchs/fastats/bodymeas.htm (accessed September 10, 2012).

CHAPTER FOUR
KICKING UP SOME DUST

1. The Harvard Medical School Family Health Guide, "Is It Okay to Be Fat if You Are Fit?", http://www.health.harvard.edu/fhg/updates/update0505c.shtml (accessed September 13, 2012).

CHAPTER SIX
BUILDING SUPPORT ON A BUDGET

1. Gary Chapman, *The Five Love Languages* (Chicago: The Northfield Publishing, 1992).

2. Mary Huizinga, Lisa Cooper, Sara Bleich, et. al., "Physician Respect for Patients With Obesity," *Journal of General Internal Medicine* 24, no. 11 (November 2009): 1236–1239.

CHAPTER EIGHT
WATCHING YOUR WALLET GET FATTER

1. National Public Radio, "The Family Dinner Deconstructed," February 25, 2008, http://www.npr.org/templates/story/story.php?storyId=19331759 (accessed September 11, 2012).

2. Zagat Survey Summary, "2012 America's Top Restaurants," http://www.zagat.com/sites/default/files/ATR12Stat%20FINAL.pdf (accessed September 11 2012).

3. Vanessa O'Connell, "Don't Get Cheated by Supermarket Scanners" *MONEY*, April 1993, http://money.cnn.com/magazines/moneymag/moneymag_archive/1993/04/01/87944/index.htm (accessed September 13, 2012).

4. American Diabetes Association, "Economic Costs of Diabetes in the U.S. in 2007," *Diabetes Care* 31, no. 3 (March 2008): 596–615.

5. Ibid

6. Ibid

7. Gregory A. Nichols, Timothy J. Bell, Kathryn L. Pedula, and Maureen O'Keefe-Rosetti, "Medical Care Costs Among Patients With Established Cardiovascular Disease," *American Journal of Managed Care* 16, no. 3 (March 2010): e86–e93; http://www.ajmc.com/articles/AJMC_10marNicholsWebX_e86to93 (accessed October 19, 2012).

8. Ibid.

9. Center to Reduce Cancer Health Disparities, *Economic Costs of Cancer Health Disparities*, US Department of Health and Human Services, http://crchd.cancer.gov/attachments/NCIeconomiccosts.pdf (accessed September 12, 2012).

CHAPTER NINE
LOSING WEIGHT LIKE A GROWN-UP

1. Thinkexist.com, "Ellen Glasgow quotes," http://thinkexist.com/quotation/the_only_difference_between_a_rut_and_a_grave_are/185387.html (accessed September 12, 2012).

2. A. N. Gearhardt, S. Yokum, P. T. Orr, et. al., "Neural Correlates of Food Addiction," *Archives of General Psychology* 68, no. 8 (August 2011): 808–816.

3. Maura Kelly, "Should 'Fatties' Get a Room? (Even on TV)," *Marie Claire*, October 25, 2010, www.marieclaire.com.

4. Ibid.

5. Ibid.

6. Max Lucado, *If I Only Had a Green Nose* (Wheaton, IL: Crossway Books, 2002).

CHAPTER TEN
TAKING YOUR PLAN ON THE ROAD

1. *When Harry Met Sally*, directed by Rob Steiner (Beverly Hills, CA: MGM, 1989), DVD.

2. Thinkexist.com, "Socrates quotes," http://thinkexist.com/quotation/worthless_people_love_only_to_eat_and_drink/297808.html (accessed September 12, 2012).

3. Jack A. Yanovski, "Holiday Weight Gain Slight, But May Last a Lifetime," National Institutes of Health, March 22, 2000, http://www.nih.gov/news/pr/mar2000/nichd-22.htm (accessed September 12, 2012).

4. Ibid.

5. Ibid.

6. Matthew 25:23, NKJV.

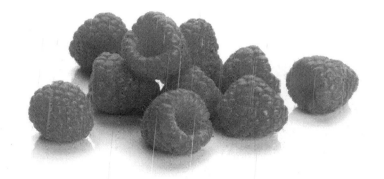

A Healthy Life—
body, mind, and spirit—
IS PART OF GOD'S PURPOSE FOR YOU!

Siloam brings you books, e-books, and other media from trusted authors on today's most important health topics. Check out the following links for more books from specialists such as *New York Times* best-selling author Dr. Don Colbert and get on the road to great health.

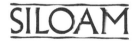

www.charismahouse.com

twitter.com/charismahouse • facebook.com/charismahouse